Bangkok Haircut

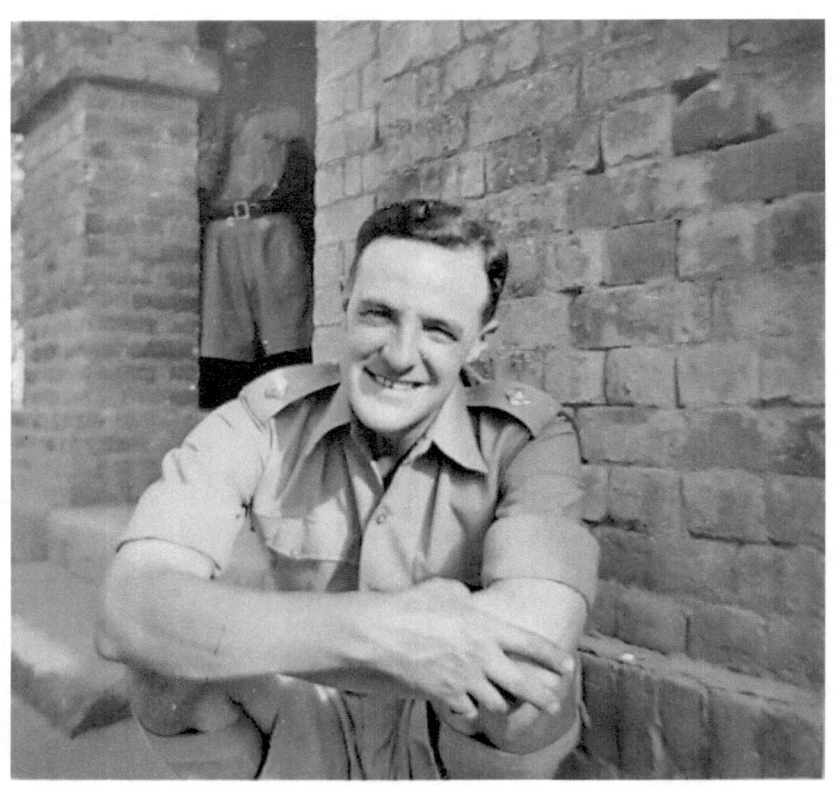

Alistair Cumming Fraser (1903-2000), circa 1943

Bangkok Haircut:
Adventures of a Veterinary Veteran

~

by Alistair Cumming Fraser LVO
QHVS PhD BVSc MRCVS

edited by Mike Fraser

Privately published

2017

First published in Great Britain in 2017

1 3 5 7 9 10 8 6 4 2

A CIP catalogue record for this book is available from the British Library

ISBN 978 1 5413 5998 7

Table of Contents

Illustrations

Introduction

Alistair Cumming Fraser was a remarkable man, a raconteur extraordinaire, who could hold any small gathering entranced with stories from his life.

Alistair was the youngest son of the actuary Duncan Cumming Fraser and Sophie née Storrar a schoolteacher who was daughter in a family of veterinary surgeons. He had a classical education, but his great love was to accompany his Uncles and Cousins on their Veterinary rounds in the holidays. When he joined Liverpool University Veterinary School, he had more experience of practical Veterinary Medicine than most of his Lecturers. At that time, Veterinary work was entirely equine. Horses were the beasts of burden, means of transport and leisure. However, as tractors were increasingly used, Alistair branched out to service racing stables and the leisure market. His veterinary life ranged from the potato fields of East Anglia to the Royal Mews at Buckingham Palace.

The Frasers at Wrexham, the Storrars at Chester and the Barrons at Little Sutton were all Scottish Presbyterians, families run along disciplinarian lines, abiding by parental wishes. Alistair signed The Teetotal Pledge aged five years at his mother's insistence. He explained that she watched the Birkenhead dockers go straight to the Public Houses on payday, and their seemingly destitute families go without for the rest of the week. Alistair never served alcohol when his parents or aunts visited, but he enjoyed a glass of sherry with his wife most evenings.

Alistair's stories include time spent in the Pasteur Institute in Paris, where he studied Equine Blood Analysis. When Alistair's son Duncan visited the Compton Research Institute in Berkshire decades later, he was astonished to learn that Alistair's blood analysis was still the standard against which all animal blood samples were measured. The work was hugely important for a generation of researchers.

Alistair described the time he spent in Burma and India during the Second World War in the Veterinary Corps as "the best time in my life". As far as he was concerned, being freed of all earthly responsibilities, with all his worldly goods in his kit bag, at one with the creatures around him, was paradise. As we discover in these stories, his life was saved by being ordered to travel across India using rudimentary transport of every kind, to attend what turned out to be a senior officer's misdiagnosis of an outbreak of swine fever. On Alistair's return he found that everyone in his Unit had been slaughtered by the Japanese.

Much of Alistair's success was due to an enquiring and analytical mind, a gentleness of spirit and an acute attention to detail. He loved his horses, whether pets or working animals. He had a huge admiration for his mules that learned so quickly to cope with the long sea journey, kettled on board all the way from South America, to being in harness, hauling huge loads of Army supplies along mountain tracks, traversing flimsy swing bridges and staying calm through gun fire. But Alistair also loved people and elicited respect and admiration in all he met, from the lowliest groom on a garden plot to the Queen Mother at the Royal Mews. In fact, he always thought that grooms were the greatest source of help and advice at any veterinary consultation. After all, they knew the animal better than anyone.

As a child, I would try to avoid Grandpa's stories, suffering from the common curse that shared inter-generational interests often come too late to be properly expressed. I had heard the best stories a multitude of times, especially as mild dementia crept up in his 90s. However, my regrets at not showing more of an interest at the time are moderated by the fact that many of his stories were documented for posterity by my grandfather himself, by my father and by Poppy Curnow, a Liverpool University researcher interested in changes in Veterinary Medicine throughout the 20th Century. Special thanks are due to them and what is presented here is mostly based on their recordings, though errors remain mine. With some trepidation, I have tried to assemble these various transcribed versions into a coherent narrative. This has required adding a few words for intelligibility or continuity and merging many duplicated stories told in different styles and with different phrasings into a whole. I have also had to sequence the stories, which are presented here in approximate order of Alistair's life, although I have had to improvise in places where historical indicators are not present. I should also thank my mum Janet Fraser who helped encourage me to work on this version and write this introduction.

Alistair had an engaging, self-deprecating way of telling his tales. I hope you will still be able to hear these qualities in his voice and appreciate them as much as I now do, too late for us to reflect together but still in time to enjoy and remember.

Mike Fraser, 6th September 2017

PART 1 – Education

Early Life

My paternal Grandfather, James Fraser was born into a crofting family in Lethendry, near Carrbridge in Inverness-shire. My maternal Grandfather, James Storrar's family kept a general store in Peterhead, Aberdeenshire, so both could genuinely claim to be Highlanders. Unknown to each other, they both looked south for employment.

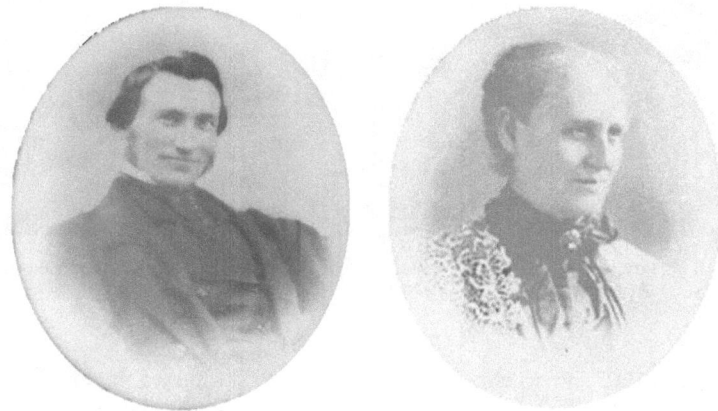

James Fraser (1833-1925) and his wife Mary née Cumming

James Fraser, hearing of a vacancy with a tailor and tea merchant in Wrexham, North Wales, took a ferry from Inverness to Oban, then walked the rest of the way to Wrexham, where he became assistant to the tailor and tea merchant. It must have been to his liking, because there he stayed. He rose to control the tailoring business, then sent home for his girlfriend Mary Cumming to come and marry him[1]. They had five sons, followed by three daughters. The eldest boy Duncan Cumming Fraser became my father.

Concurrently, James Storrar was sent to a veterinary college in Glasgow to qualify, and James and his particular college friend Will Barron married Morrison sisters and joined or created veterinary practices in Chester and Little Sutton, five miles from each other. The Storrars in Chester raised five sons and four daughters, the eldest girl Sophia Storrar became my mother. She was a schoolteacher.

Two Fraser brothers married two Storrar sisters – Duncan Cumming Fraser married Sophie Storrar, and Alexander 'Alec' Fraser married Cecelia Jessie Storrar, the latter couple without issue. Neil Barron married Annie Storrar, Sophie's Aunt and the Barrons raised a large family.

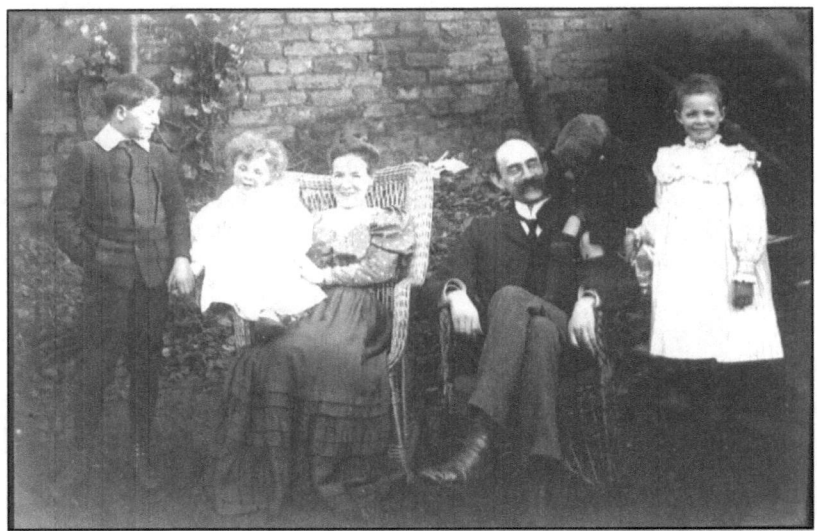

Frasers in Birkenhead (left to right): Lesley, Alistair, Sophie, Duncan, Neil (leaning over his father's shoulder, barely visible) and Margaret

I was born in 1903 in Birkenhead on Merseyside, aware from my cradle that my ambition was to be a veterinary surgeon for horses. My father[2], a mathematician who had been a Cambridge wrangler, was The Royal Insurance Company's actuary in Liverpool. He and his family had no veterinary interests, nor had my brothers and sisters. My two brothers' and two sisters' interests were in medicine and Christian missions. My mother[3] had been a school teacher but, significantly, she was a vet's daughter. I have always been grateful to my mother that she transmitted that essential gene to me. My maternal Grandfather James Storrar[4] was a veterinary surgeon, but he died at eighty, when I was five and I remember him only vaguely by his purple and gold skull cap. He had a veterinary practice in Chester and his family tree was so well endowed with vets that I never had any ambition other than to become a veterinary surgeon.

I am told I was a puny child, but the care of my mother and my six childless aunts pulled me through. I was a consumptive child with a persistent cough. I followed my brothers, who were two and five years older to Birkenhead school. I was accepted at the age of five as a day boy to the preparatory section, with a note from my doctor suggesting that I should be excused from homework and games. This was agreed, so until I left the 'Prep' at ten and moved to the senior school, I was cosseted by these concessions. In my school holidays, and when I was not robust enough to go to school, I was regularly packed off to my aunts who pampered a rather frail nephew and let me run wild in North Wales. Their kindness and the bracing air helped me to over-whelm my consumption, and I developed my own interests: natural history or pottering about rather aimlessly (but taking it all in), and horses.

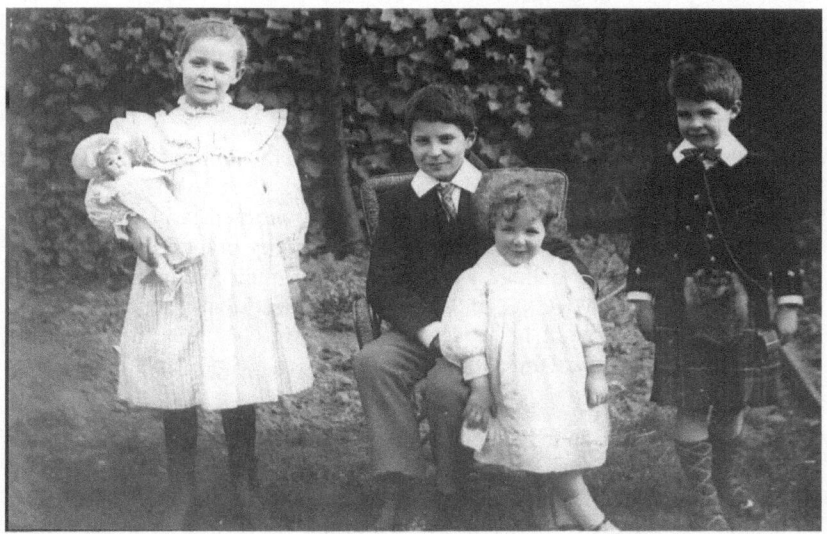

Frasers in Birkenhead (left to right): Margaret, Lesley, Alistair and Neil

With my promotion to the senior school, as I had lost my cough and was in reasonable health, I expected that I would become 'normal' and be expected to take part in games and do my homework like my brothers, but it seems my doctor's note of five years before had been passed on, on the top of my file! Who was to dispute my doctor's orders? I might have felt a pariah, especially as getting no marks for homework meant I was bottom of all the weekly class lists. Actually, I was delighted to keep a low profile and enjoy my lavish spare time.

As my brothers had taken classics at School, so did I. My sisters, both para-gons of virtue, finding I was ambitious to be educated and that I enjoyed writ-ing and was good at languages, decided they would assist me to educate myself. Aware that I couldn't pass exams unaided, they took my case seri-ously and advised me that, as I was incapable of remembering anything I was taught, my only chance of passing exams was to consider the question, mull over it to detect a slight response, and then write an original answer that was interesting (they knew I could do that!) even though it had no relevance to the original questions. Suicidal! But I got through exams. They said it was because it was such a relief to the examiner to get away from the routine of correct answers, that they would forgive me for misreading the questions and give me a pass mark for luck.

The outbreak of war against Germany in 1914 rather broke up our family. My brother Lesley was called up for military service[5] and my sisters[6] became involved in foreign missions but I was too young to be included. However, aged eleven years, I stayed on in Birkenhead School and became an Army Cadet with the Cadet Corps, Cheshire Regiment until I left school in 1922, Rank: Lance Corporal. We drilled and marched and learned to shoot with rifles, and camped under canvas for ten days or a fortnight each summer.

At My Uncles' Veterinary Practices

My mother was a veterinary surgeon's daughter, so I was not entirely unaware of what I was letting myself in for when I decided, as quite a small boy, that I would like to be a veterinary surgeon too. My mother had two brothers[7], two uncles, and three cousins who were in veterinary practice. They had all been sent to veterinary college without option by their Victorian veterinary fathers to qualify as MRCVS, and they were amazed that I actually wanted to be a vet. They thought I was cracked. They weren't alone in that, but I really soaked up clinical information over the ten years I spent time with them.

To keep me occupied in my school holidays when war broke out, my mother sent me to stay with one or other of her veterinary relatives in Dorset, Wiltshire, Berkshire, and South Wales, who generously put me up and let me sit alongside as they drove or were driven in their traps or gigs as they were attending to their clients' horses. They never tried to teach me anything or explain what they were doing, but I was welcome to watch or talk to the owners, grooms or stable boys as much as I liked. I had regular sessions seeing how my uncles treated horses from the time I was eleven until I became an undergraduate at the Liverpool university veterinary college at the age of eighteen.

While I was at school, my father got a book from a lending library written by two American vets in which they stated that "no odium attached itself amongst the general public to false statement made in support of the sale of a horse". This open declaration of the acceptance of the dishonesty of horse dealing really impressed me and I made a personal and private declaration to myself (not being above telling a lie now and again to get myself out of trouble) that as regards horses (and it was veterinary work with horses that I was aiming at), I would report them as I found them, and I believe I have done this ever since, in spite of offers of bribes and some nerve-shattering threats. I could never have established the reputation I wanted if I had ever deviated from this resolve.

In those days, vets attended horses. Horses were in great variety, heavy horses for farm work and to pull lorries, lighter horses for buses, trams and commercial deliveries, cabs and hunting, down to ponies pulling traps and for children to ride: from Shires at a ton to Shetland ponies at two hundred lbs. With the ancillary interest of saddlery and harness, farriers made the shoes and nailed them on. The chief reason that vets were not called to attend to sick farm animals or dogs, cats or any other pets was that they did not know and were not expected to know anything about animals other than the horse. They might help a farmer with a difficult cow calving but, apart from that, farm animals' health was the farmer's responsibility, pets were in their owner's care, while vets treated horses. The Ministry of Agriculture employed some vets to deal with outbreaks of Anthrax, Foot and Mouth disease and Swine Fever, but they were infrequent. Farmers applied simple first aid for their minor problems. More serious cases were dealt with by Knackers, who dealt with 'Fallen Stock' and provided meat for dogs: or they were sent to the Hunt kennels for the same purpose. Sick sheep just died and were buried or used as dog food, whilst pigs, one at the bottom of most village gardens remained constantly healthy in their isolation until they ended up as hams or sides hanging from the kitchen ceiling. So, early in the twentieth century a veterinary surgeon's chief interest was maintaining horses' health. Vets were beginning to include farm animals in their range and, rather tentatively, domestic pets, but horse practice was their mainstay. Vets were horse doctors and though horses were declining in the realms of transport, it was a horse doctor I wanted to be.

I emerged at the age of about sixteen and started to pass exams and gained confidence. Around this time, I was associating frequently with Clifford Hall-Jones, who was working with his father in Liverpool as a tailor[8]. I was lucky to be allowed to see a variety of different Veterinary Practices. Uncle David Storrar in South Wales kept an eye on hundreds of working ponies working the coal mines, Uncle James 'Jim' Storrar added farm horses, hunters and polo ponies in Cheshire, and cousin Will Barron in Lambourn, Wiltshire attended the horses at thirty or forty racing stables and several stud farms.

Whenever I could, I went to stay with Uncle Robert 'Bob' Barron[9] in Blandford, Dorset who attended general practice including a wide range of horses on large estates and a variety of riding horses in the Bournemouth area. I soon found that Uncle Bob was of uncertain temper, traceable to chronic indigestion for which he blamed his father, also a veterinary surgeon, who had forced him into the profession against his will and kept him so short of money while he was a student that he couldn't afford adequate nourishment. I wasn't at all sure how justified his self-pity was but, as long as I kept my mouth shut, I got by and, in a way, I think Uncle Bob enjoyed my company. He almost seemed pleased when I turned up again and again.

I told him one day that I was hoping to become a vet. I thought it would have been obvious but, according to my aunt, the idea surprised him and he determined to put an end to such nonsense by letting me in on the really seamy side of veterinary practice: pain, misery, suffering, cruelty and death. He wasn't much of a psychologist! I didn't notice any marked changes of emphasis in relationship with my uncle as I was continually widening my experiences and accepting more responsibilities and we continued on good terms even when he employed an assistant. He was not destined to retire. His illnesses got worse and he died suddenly at work. We had different attitudes but I was glad we never quarrelled. I was able to assist his assistant for a while, but I left as I had further training in mind.

Ten Riding Lessons for £5

When I was staying with my Uncle Bob in Dorset in my early teens, and he knew I wanted to be a vet, he was quite surprised to find that I couldn't ride. Vetting, to him, meant horses. He arranged for me to help the local hunt to exercise their horses doing daily, walking and trotting in the Dorset lanes for a couple of hours to get them "muscled up" for the approaching winter hunting season. I didn't have to do anything except just sit on the saddled horse passively while the horse, one of a string of ten or eleven, walked or trotted with the rest. The exercise was passive for me as all I had to do was to sit there, but it was agony for my muscles and joints which had to adjust to the increasing activity. I did that daily for 3 weeks and it took about as long as that again for me to lose the aches and pains. Though I have done a lot of riding since, I have never had the same discomfort again – the necessary adjustments were adequate and permanent.

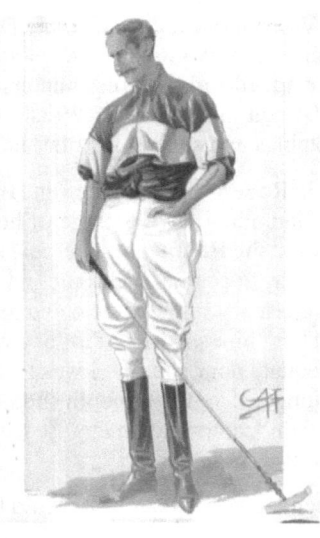

Caricature of Mike Rimington taken from Vanity Fair, 1898

Riding was essential to their assessment of a horse's health and condition, and I became increasingly conscious of the fact that I still could not ride well. In my late 'teens I raised this point with my father. He found a notice in the local paper advertising ten riding lessons for five pounds, and he suggested that I should make my own enquiries.

The stables were at Parkgate, by the shore of the Dee estuary, six miles from where we lived in Birkenhead, so no problem to me on my bike. I met Captain Mike Rimington[10], who had just retired from the army Remounts[11], the 1914-18 war being over. He had about twenty polo ponies that he let out to members of the Hooton Polo Club which was about five miles from the stables. Riding lessons were his wife's idea. I liked the air of efficient horsemanship in an otherwise casual atmosphere and handed over my father's five pounds.

When I told Mike of my requirements he said he was too busy to give me a lesson just then, but he put me up on a polo pony, gave me a stick and a ball and told me to knock the ball about on the sands for a bit which were about a couple of hundred yards away from the stables. I did that, put down the ball, swiped at it and fell off. Fortunately, sand makes comfortable landing and the pony trotted back to the stables, where I was remounted and went back to the sands, only to fall off again and so on. Polo pony is rather a misnomer. They are mostly as high as a horse and only called ponies because no-one talks about polo horses. To a tyro, especially a small one, a polo pony's saddle is a long way up. So, Mike said I'd better spend the rest of the lesson practising mounting. The other lesson to be learned was jumping – both mounting and jumping needed practice. Getting off wasn't difficult using gravity, but getting on needed help for a long time. As I got taller and a little stronger, I could manage better. I spent any spare time I could find helping at the Rimington's pony stables. I never got any riding lessons as such, however I got on so well with the Rimingtons and their ponies that I received many times £5-worth of interest and experience,

On one occasion, I went with Mike on his motor bike and sidecar to see a pony in Northwich (or was it Nantwich?) he thought of buying. He was shown the pony and rode it using his own saddle and bridle from the sidecar. It was what he required so he bought the pony and asked me to ride it back to Parkgate for him. I was delighted to be given the responsibility of riding a valuable pony, and I set off at a trot for Chester. It hadn't seemed far on the motor bike and the pony and I got on well for the first five miles. My enthusiasm waned a little when the pony decided that enough was enough and turned back for his home stable. I broke a switch out of the hedge with some difficulty, unwilling to dismount as I was not sure that I would be able to get back to the saddle again. The stick persuaded my mount to trot another few miles in my chosen direction, but anxiety for his next meal overwhelmed him and he refused to go any further from home. A signpost showed it was another eight miles to Chester and I knew that Parkgate was about ten miles beyond that. So I had to get off and walk. I was thankful that he agreed to be led. We plodded on. Daylight and my enthusiasm faded away together, if we could maintain our sad pace of about three miles an hour we might get there by midnight. I was usually fairly good at wriggling out of awkward situations, so I put this one to my subconscious mind to mull over while we plodded on. I thought of the AA, the RSPCA. and the Red Cross but, alas: no vehicle, no cruelty, and no blood to justify their roles.

I thought I could find my cousin's veterinary yard in Chester and I thought he might accommodate me and the pony for the night. I was related vaguely to vets all over the country; and there was a family of them in Chester, and I had once been to the house; though I didn't know which generation was functioning. However, I recalled that, in the proper Victorian tradition, my teetotal grandfather had forbidden his veterinary son to marry the rich brewer's daughter and, when his son disobeyed, grandfather not finding it convenient to throw his son out, indicated his umbrage by returning to Wales with most of his daughters including my mother who dutifully severed contact with her erring brother.

The pony was a drag but, like a drowning man clutching at straws, we made it. I prepared myself for a rebuff from my cousin which would mean walking until midnight. At about 8 o'clock I turned into the yard in Watergate Street. Cousin Jim had heard the horse coming down the street and hospitably agreed to provide a stable for the pony and supper and a bed for me. He accommodated the horse first, in a horse box with hay and water, and then took me in for tea and toast. I asked him if I might ring home to ease my mother's mind. He said "Help yourself. The 'phone is just by you." She hadn't even noticed that I wasn't around! My cousin commented "Now I know who you are." He had presumed that I was a relative and had already warned his assistant that he would have to move over in bed for a few hours. After breakfast, he pointed me toward Parkgate and gave the pony a whack on the quarter that set me off at a good pace that I was able to maintain. I was very grateful for the hospitality but only gradually began to understand that my troubles were not of real concern to anyone but myself, a view which was confirmed on my arrival back at Parkgate.

Both the Captain and his wife were out; the stable staff accepted the arrival of yet another pony, and I got on my bicycle and rode home. I cycled over a few days later to fix up about lessons, but Mike was too busy to give me one just then. As it was a polo day, they would be glad of my help in hacking some of the ponies to Hooton and back. I would have appreciated a 'Thanks' or 'How did you get on?' but, with twenty ponies to organise, one safe delivery went un-noticed. I continued to help them ferry ponies on the five-mile trips to and from the Hooton Club ground, riding one and leading one or even two others during three polo seasons.

I was able to help Mike with a problem after I qualified as a vet, simply by persuading him to go ahead with a case. He had offered a pony to a titled gentleman whose son wanted to play polo at Cambridge. Sir D., himself a polo player put the pony through the full routine of a veterinary examination, approved the pony and bought it for £250. The pony was sent to Cambridge where it was found to be lame and on a Cambridge Veterinary surgeon's advice was put down as suffering from incurable arthritis. Sir D. sued Mike Rimington for selling him an unsound pony. The Cambridge vet and I had some parleying over technicalities, but I did not play a significant part in the judgement that was delivered. After Mike had been asked what he had paid for the pony, Mike enquired if he had to answer the question? He was told that he must, and he said "£25". The judgement duly delivered was to the effect that if Sir D. considered that he knew so much about horses that he could do without a veterinary surgeon's opinion, and he had made what proved to be a full veterinary examination on his own behalf and found the horse suitable for his purposes, he must abide by his own conclusions. So Mike won his case! I have been interested to read from time to time that Sir D.'s bombast has continued to involve him in scandalous situations.

Liverpool

At the age of 19, I became an undergraduate at the Liverpool University's Veterinary School. I had been led to suppose that the veterinary section of Liverpool University had an annual entry of thirty to forty students. In 1921 there were eight of us, and one of those was a girl! What had happened was that cars and tractors were replacing horses at such a rate that it was accepted that the need would be for more mechanics and very few young people thought of devoting their lives to horses. The general view was that a veterinary career was doomed.

We were so few in the intake that we were lumped together with medical and dental students for everything except anatomy, which was confined to the horse. The basic sciences: botany, zoology, physiology, chemistry and physics were all very well taught. The university had a specialised department, headed by a professor, in each of these subjects. They were new to me as I had been in the classics stream at school. I was glad of the arrangement as I was lucky to make friends amongst my fellow students who had taken chemistry and physics at school and were prepared to coach me in what I found to be very difficult subjects. Helping me relieved them of some of the boredom of having to attend lectures on familiar themes.

This left anatomy to be varied according to group interests which, for veterinary students I was glad to see, was still the horse. These were all items that were essential to a proper understanding of clinical cases to which we advanced in later terms: medicine, surgery, farriery and lameness, all of major importance in relation to horses, though maximum attention was given to soundness, which covers the whole usefulness of a horse, not only its freedom from lameness. A sound horse is free from any condition that does or might reduce the usefulness of the animal for the purpose for which it was being acquired. When the examination is being made in connection with the sale of an animal, it is up to the purchaser to instruct and pay for a veterinary surgeon to examine the horse and find it to be sound, if that is his conclusion. A certificate of soundness from the vendor's vet, if there was to be any dispute, is not considered to be a viable document: simply because the pressure to favour a payee is liable to affect any judgement. The veterinary schools went very thoroughly into these questions of lameness and soundness. The big question seemed to be – would there be enough horses to keep the veterinary profession in existence.

Practical classes for the veterinary students were carried out on the carriage horses that pulled the hearses in the Undertaker's stables down the road from the Liverpool Veterinary College. The clinical teaching was not of a high standard. There were far more medical and dental faculty students than veterinary ones, so the lecturers and examiners were usually familiar with dosages and methods applicable to human patients, rather than horses and cattle. When I could, I led the questioning to horse and cattle dosages, such as 1½ lb. of Epsom Salts by stomach tube to a constipated cow! They just goggled! But I maintained that the enormous dosages I had mentioned were based on cases that I had attended and I rather implied that I doubted if they had ever seen a constipated cow. They hadn't much of a leg to stand on! I was quoting clinical practice against their ignorance because, thanks to my uncles, not only had I seen the cases but I'd administered the medicines too.

I qualified as an MRCVS, a Member of the Royal College of Veterinary Surgeons, in 1926. My health was much improved and I was enjoying being an undergraduate so I stayed on a few more terms to take the BVSc degree, Bachelor of Veterinary Science. During my time at Liverpool I spent some time seeing practice with James White MRCVS in Sefton Park, who also had a farriery business with 4 anvils, and also with Charles Elam[12] who dealt with the heavy horses servicing the Merseyside docks and traffic. My uncles also continued to let me spend my university vacations with one or other of them until I started in practice myself.

I got through on ignorance and ingenuity, and one of the professors directed my interests towards horses' blood cells and their variations and diseases. I so impressed Professor Geiger[13] that he arranged for the Ministry of Agriculture to award me a scholarship to stay on and help him investigate equine haematology and blood diseases of horses. I amused myself by supposing it was mistaken identity! This was influenced by the fact he himself was suffering from recurrent Surra[14], with which he had been infected in India. I was arranging to assist one of my veterinary uncles, when I had a letter from The Ministry regretting Professor Geiger's death and instructing me to report to a Professor Buxton in Cambridge.

Cambridge

While I still had two years to put in at Liverpool University, I continued to cycle over to Parkgate when I had time to spare and usually got involved in ferrying ponies to and from the Hooton ground. I enjoyed the riding and watching the polo and I got quite a few chukkas of polo just to fill in if they were short. Three players and a novice were better than three against four.

After the professor under whom I was to study died suddenly, the Ministry of

Agriculture decided that my further training was to be at Cambridge. I left full of gratitude to the Parkgate family for letting me acquire a familiarity with horses that has been invaluable to me ever since, even though the boss was always too busy, just then, to give me every one of the ten lessons my father had paid for. I had bought one of their polo ponies for eight pounds. It was blind in one eye and so was barred from polo, but it gave me great satisfaction to have my own pony to ride. I never got very good at polo but I could refer to it casually, and even mention my own pony's behaviour, when I felt my social status: but that had to be used very cautiously.

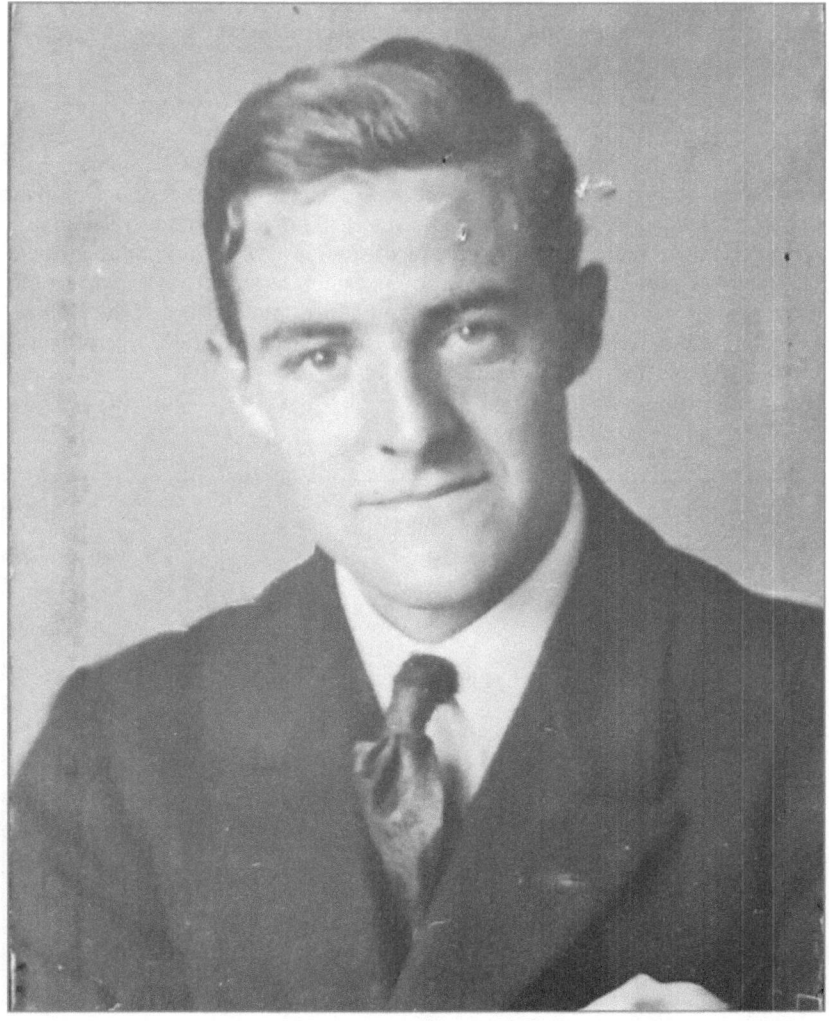

Alistair in 1927

In 1927 I reported to Professor Buxton[15] at the Cambridge University Field Laboratories. Professor Buxton's veterinary staff were investigating farm animal diseases. The laboratory was also producing quantities of equine blood serum as a diluent for medical vaccines. However, as this Organisation was attached to Cambridge University, Buxton said he was only allowed to accept students who were in a Cambridge college and with regret he would not be able to admit me. I casually I remarked that I was sorry too, but my father would be even more so as he was ex-Trinity Hall and a mathematical Wrangler at that College. This immediately rendered me eligible for entry to Trinity Hall and the Field Laboratories! He suggested that I should make a study of blood cells and their variants as my subject.

I asked Prof Buxton if he could accommodate a polo pony to which he agreed. Horses being then commonly carried by train; a friend took my pony with its saddle and bridle to the railway station at Birkenhead and I collected it at Cambridge station later in the day and rode it to the Field Laboratories. The department where I was to study had a stable of horses which were available for veterinary research and my director of studies agreed to fit another horse in. I had not thought that the arrival of an undergraduate with his own polo pony would even be noticed in the generally elitist atmosphere of the University, but I was offered membership of the University Polo Club, which I gathered was expensive. I couldn't afford it anyway but I joined the Cambridgeshire hunt[16].

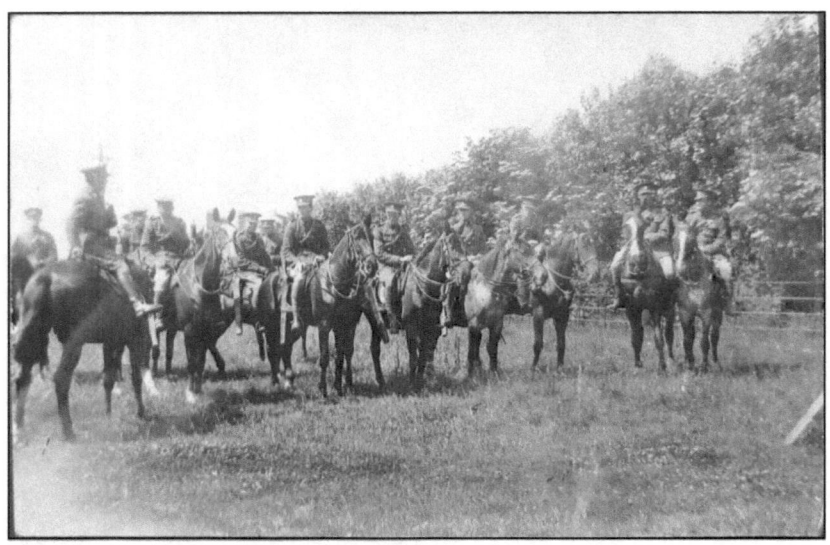

Territorials in Cambridge led by the unimpressed Major Cooper, 1928

I was also expected to link up with the Cambridgeshire Regiment, which still at that time had a small horse squadron, for regular parades and an annual camp. However, as the Territorial Army quite correctly had no record of my receiving riding instruction, I was required to report to the leading riding school in Cambridge run by a Major Cooper, to assess my fitness to be classed as a Trooper. Major Cooper was not impressed – I had not expected him to be. But I was thankful, at long last to be put through a thoroughly professional course of equitation to cavalry standard that was of the utmost benefit to me for many years.

I seemed to have two problems: firstly, could I find time to fit in all these commitments together with my academic studies; and secondly, could I meet the expenses involved. As horsemanship was my primary ambition, I determined to fit in all the training I could. That left me to add up the outlay. I found that my pony was listed as an experimental animal (together with the white mice and beagle puppies), so stabling and the attention of a groom were paid for by the University. Hunt membership was free to undergraduates.; and if I took Major Cooper's full course of riding instruction and fitted in the annual fortnight's camp, these items would be charged to the Army. So, the cost to me would be nil.

Unfortunately, my pony's blind eye cost him his life. I was riding on the tow path by the river Cam when a pheasant rose at the pony's feet with the usual explosive clattering call. The pony shied to the right, his blind side, and we both ended up in the river. I had gone over the animal's head, taking the reins with me. The reins got caught up in the pony's feet and he never got his head above water. I replaced him with a hunter gelding to see me through my second year, after which I was transferred to work at the Pasteur Institute in Paris, and gave up riding for a while.

I continued my study of equine haematology with some interruptions as Professor Buxton asked me to attend the Annual General Meeting of the British Association for the Advancement of Science of which he was a member. He was too busy to attend it and I could have his ticket if I liked. I wasn't at all keen to join what the dictionary defined as "philosophical discussions not generally intelligible", but I had to show some interest in Buxton's kind offer. The meeting was to take place in Cape Town and Pretoria. This was 1930. In those days one didn't hop on a plane. One went on a liner to Cape Town and by train to Pretoria, then back by another liner up the African East Coast and back through the Mediterranean. Expeditions filled the month of August very enjoyably and I managed to fit in a visit to one of my father's brothers (Uncle Alec Fraser) who was a stock inspector in the Durban area and I was able to spend a few days at the South African Veterinary Research laboratory whose Director I had met some time ago when he was on a visit to England.

On returning to Cambridge I was continuing my investigations into equine leukaemia, but Professor Buxton told me he had booked me a place on a course for medical and veterinary research workers at the Pasteur Institute in Paris for 6 months, from October to March.

A Winter in Paris

When I got back from attending the British Association's meetings in South Africa, Professor Buxton told me that the Pasteur Institute in Paris had a vacancy on an advanced course they were conducting for veterinary research workers and that he had put my name forward. The course, from October to March, sounded as though it was exactly what I required, and I was pleased to hear shortly that I had been accepted.

With help from one of my sisters, who had spent some time in Paris, I found an inexpensive room not far from the Institute. With the multiplicity of catering establishments in Paris it seemed sensible that I should eat independently and I found that a great many Parisians called in somewhere for their coffee and a roll on their way to work. I settled down to the Paris routine of a short breakfast on the way to work, a two hour break for lunch, and the evenings free from 6 o'clock.

I reported to the Pasteur Institute and was directed to the office of a Professor Levaditi[17], where I was enrolled as a temporary member of his staff and introduced to his research team; an American girl, a Russian girl and a Scottish lad of about my own age. There was also a staff of three or four laboratory assistants. I was to rank as a research worker. There was no language problem as the American and the Scot soon had me chattering in French, while the Russian girl, hardly ever said anything other than 'storch', which was Russian for 'What?'.

I attended three sessions of the course I was entered for, but I soon realised that the standard was so elementary that I was unlikely to gain any benefit from it. I explained this to my research colleagues who broke the news to Professor Levaditi, who would only listen to fluent French, and it was arranged that I should proceed with the work on blood cells that I had begun at Liverpool and continued at Cambridge where I was hoping one day to become a Doctor of Philosophy. I am especially grateful to Anita Howard, the American girl, for helping me translate some of my small publications into French. Not long after that she met a British army officer who had won a Victoria Cross and they are happily married. There are not many about of that quality! I am sorry to have lost touch.

Professor Levaditi was distant, but helpful, and I earned a good mark for the quality of my blood slides, the preparation of which I had learned from my doctor and dentist Liverpool friend, Laurie Roberts, who seemed able to do most things rather better than anybody else. Levaditi was so pleased that he wrote to Professor Buxton in Cambridge to say so. I had another stroke of luck. When I arrived late at the laboratory one day and asked why such gloom, I was told that an experimental animal, a white rat, had just died, whereby the Professor had lost information vitally important to some research he had in hand. They showed me the body, still warm, I recalled my Uncle Bob's method of reviving moribund new-born calves. He had them swung 'head down'. So we swung the rat 'head down' and, like some of my uncle's calves, the rat began to breathe again and the English veterinary profession collected another good mark.

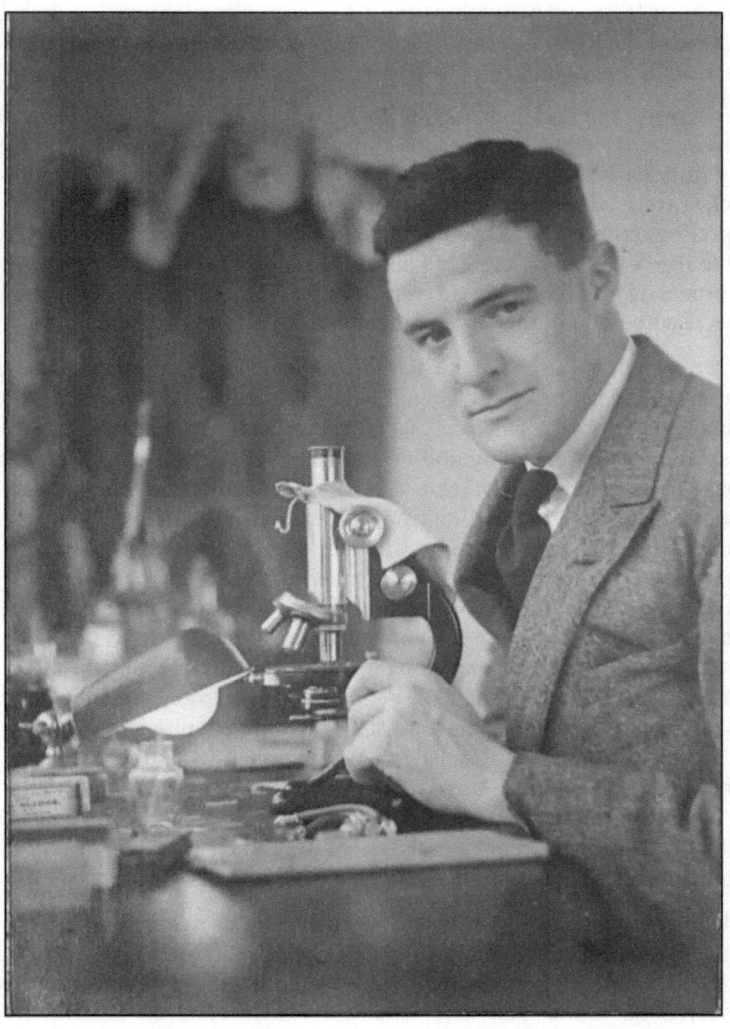

Preparing blood slides does not necessarily preclude looking suave

I had other successes. The cat at an Italian café where I lunched occasionally, took ill. Somebody told them I was a vet. I prescribed and the cat survived. Six years later I took a friend there to lunch. The cat didn't remember me, but the owners did and they insisted that the cat, still going strong, was to be charged for our very substantial meal.

In the cause of good health, I joined the British Rugby Club, which trained at the Paris Y.M.C.A. It was well worth it, even if only to see and hear the excitement any French youth could enjoy in half a minute under a cold shower. While most of our club members were British, we had a few Frenchmen and a couple of Russians who joined for the opportunity of practising their English. One of the Russians, in a friendly quarrel, threatened me with 'I kill you Fraser, I kill you twice!'.

I was surprised to find how popular rugby was in France. A great many small towns and villages had their rugby clubs. I was elected hooker. The further away from Paris the more overpowering the garlic in the scrums. At times our matches were advertised locally as 'Grandes Matches Internationales', and the preliminaries could outdo the match itself: two National Anthems, and a visit to the War Memorial being part of the routine. We took a wreath with us and produced it, if required. We were quite a popular fixture because the local teams usually won. It mattered to them and we played for the fun of it.

Our scrum-half, on a scholarship to the Sorbonne University, to promote good relations between France and Great Britain, was a gifted entertainer, choosing to sing and perform step dances on café tables with varying success. Some of the smaller places encouraged him: the larger ones, who employed professionals, threw him out. His theme song 'Les Gendarmes de Montparnasse, ils ne sont pas gentils', did not improve his relations with the police who occasionally locked him up for minor offences. He frequently changed his lodgings, always leaving word that he was moving to Moscow, but he never did. He had an extensive collection of firearms which I took to be antiques, but soon realised that they were modern and lethal; another reason for the police to keep an eye on him. He explained that his behavioural oddities helped him to understand the French social system. On one occasion, when he had been showing me his weapons and their uses with great enthusiasm, he told me he had to meet a girl at Cap Finisterre, rather urgently, and could I lend him twenty Francs to make up the rail fare as he was short of cash, which I did; and thought no more about it, until a few days later the Continental Daily Mail had a front page report on the death of the heir to a British estate, in a shooting accident. Paris has the strongest of influences.

Back to rugby football. We had two interesting matches: one against the French army cadets and one against the police. Playing the young officers, the weather was wet but bearable. We were a little ahead in the scoring when we scored again after half-time. The rain came on and we found ourselves with fewer and fewer opponents as one by one they drifted off the field. They were tall, slim and fast but, as the result was obvious, they saw no point in getting wetter. I think it is known as pragmatism! By contrast, the police team, mostly Basques from the Spanish border area, were shorter, thicker and slower than the army team, and they seemed to be blessed with three legs each, being impossible to put off balance. They beat us by a large score.

The Chinese researcher at the Pasteur Institute was a gentle character with a nice sense of humour. We took him out to lunch on somebody's birthday. The French generally take two hours for their lunch break to make up for the hasty breakfast snack. We had wine to toast the birthday and Dr Li, usually teetotal, drank with us. When we got up to go he said, rather carefully, 'I am quite well, but my legs are very drunk. I think we will stay here.' He turned up later on, when his legs had sobered up. He liked playing with words. He chuckled over a London bus conductor solemnly asking him 'Where to? China?' and he showed off his polyglot ability by telling us that if you said 'Shut t' door' to an Englishman, he would do just that; while if you said the same sounds as 'Je t'adore' to a French girl, she might slap your face! I wonder how that story would sound in Chinese!

The laboratory staff was led by a Monsieur Bernard, who was held in rather fearsome respect by all those over whom he exercised his authority, creating an atmosphere in which biological and scientific observations were para-mount and no frivolities were thought of, let alone tolerated. Having no do-mestic responsibilities or set meals, I sampled various restaurants and cafés and I was surprised now and again to come across acquaintances from Eng-land, though it was natural enough. There were students from Liverpool or Cambridge or London, on courses in Paris, and our paths were likely enough to converge eventually. It was somebody from London who told me about the rugby club at the Paris Y.M.C.A. and a young vet from Australia, whom I had met in Dorset when he was visiting my Uncle Bob, tracked me down and we did a little shopping together. It was so much more fun pottering about in Paris with somebody else than doing it alone, that I suggested to the Scottish lad on the Levaditi staff that we might do a bit of exploring together, but I got a solemn rebuff. He told me he was in Paris 'to enhance his studies'. So was I but not for twenty-four hours a day.

However, I did better. I found my guide to the lighter side of Parisian life in the person of the most unlikely candidate of all my (few) acquaintances in Paris: Monsieur Bernard!

On one of my evening expeditions pottering round in the Folies Bergère The-atre district, I saw somebody resembling him – he was in charge at a souvenir stall. He caught my eye as I recognised him and I wondered what this might lead to! He greeted me by name and introduced me with a hint of pride to his companions. When I left them, he asked me not to refer to his moonlighting at the Institute. At Monsieur Bernard's request, I kept quiet about his second occupation. Anita Howard did comment that I must have made a particular

impression on Monsieur Bernard as he was looking after my laboratory requirements so very solicitously. Through him I met quite a few Parisians and
through these introductions, and in playing rugby for the YMCA in Paris
against various small town and college teams on Saturdays and Sundays, I
really enjoyed being an Englishman in Paris. I found myself adopted into the
pleasant domesticity of native Parisian company to such an extent that I was
never at a loss, when I was not 'enhancing my studies', for interest and en-
tertainment.[18]

I hadn't gained much from my winter in Paris, except for a fluency in French,
which I have never needed since, and the opportunity to complete and write
up my blood cell thesis, which Cambridge thought adequate to justify a doc-
torate in 1930. I assumed my conclusions would then be filed away into the
oblivion of a university library. However, my son, who qualified as a vet in
1966, now tells me that my blood cell tables were quoted as authoritative in
his time at college some thirty years later, so I hadn't strained my brain altogether in vain!

Early Veterinary Practice

Following my PhD Cantab, I decided to quit academics and bought what was
left of a veterinary practice in the Boston and Skegness area, where we
worked with heavy horses working the rich soil of the potato fields. The vet
running the practice had died and his veterinary son, released from his father's restraint, took up drinking seriously and soon joined his father. I bought
what was left of the goodwill for a few hundred pounds and Clifford Hall-
Jones, my friend from Birkenhead days joined me to help run the practice.

Within a few years (1930-1933) however, a bright engineer flogged mechanical horse power to all the potato farmers, and all I had left to treat was a
number of Skegness domestic pets, which remnant was taken over for a pit-
tance by a Boston firm.

In 1933 I bought my Uncle Will Barron's share of the Lambourn practice for
£3,000 as he wanted to break away from his "dead slow" partner Eric Gill
and I wanted to treat thoroughbred horses in the racing stables and stud farms.
Uncle Will knew of a group of doctors who were in business dealing in medical instruments and he bought a share to extend that to include veterinary
instruments with my £3,000. He never heard from them again – a bit of a
shock, but he was relieved to be rid of partner Gill.

Gill was hopeless – so thorough that he could average 2 or 3 cases a day, but
he was bearable to me as my entrée to thoroughbreds. So, I ignored him and
was really building up a rapidly expanding Practice amongst the numerous
racing stables using the Lambourn, Marlborough and White Horse Hill gallops. However, the 1939-45 war stopped all horse racing.

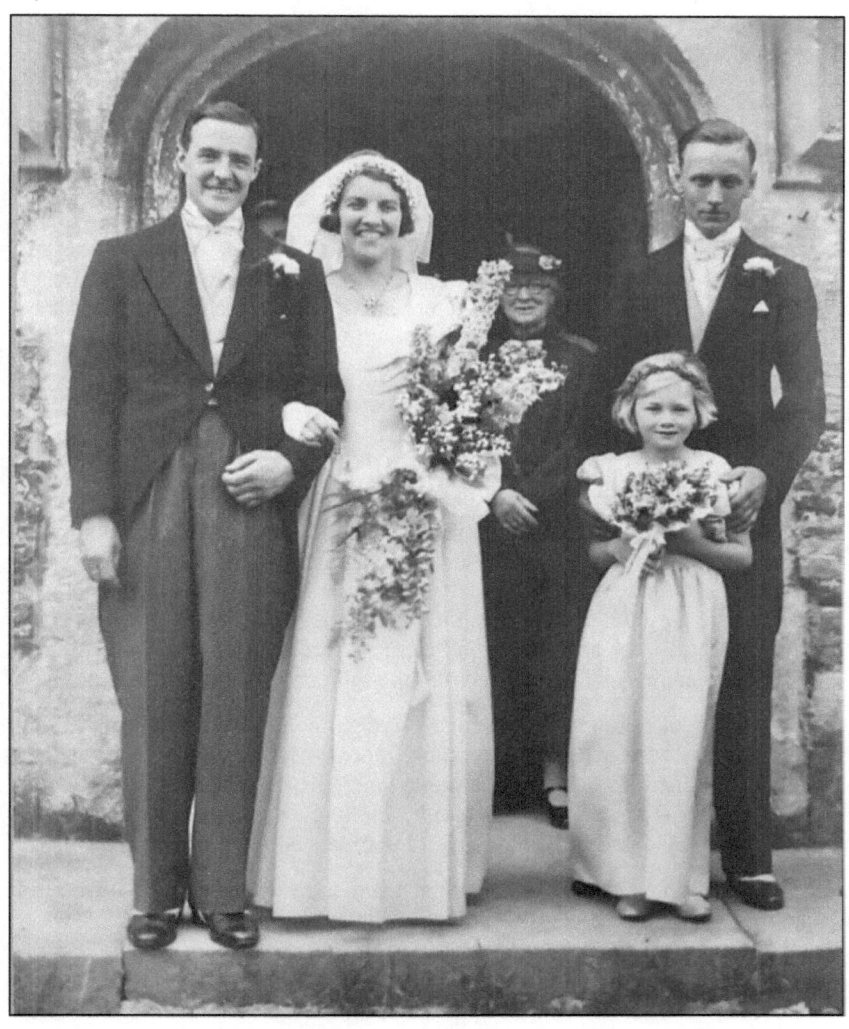

Alistair married Olive née Purver in Hungerford, 1935 [19]

Part 2 – The Army

The Army

When war was declared against Germany in 1914, I was eleven years old. I was at Birkenhead School and the school formed a cadet corps as part of the Cheshire Regiment which we all joined, parading regularly on Fridays in khaki uniform to be drilled and marched and taught to shoot with rifles. The war ended four years later in 1918 but the cadet corps continued and in 1921, when I was eighteen and a Lance Corporal, I was transferred to the Liverpool University Territorials branch of the Royal Lancashire Regiment and occasionally continued to be drilled and marched at a few parades and got in some shooting practice, mostly during our annual fortnight summer camp.

When, four years later at the age of twenty-four, I was moved again to Cambridge and the army discovered that I had my own horse. I was transferred to a squadron, still horsed, of the Cambridgeshire regiment's mounted squadron whose annual fortnight of camp was inclined to resemble a gymkhana and was thoroughly enjoyable. I found that I was required to take a full course of military riding instruction, including jumping, up to the standard required of all mounted officers, for which the army sent us to the leading riding school in Cambridge under Major Cooper. I moved to Paris and my territorial military service lapsed, though I remained in their records. I then had a few years of agricultural work and then switched most successfully to work for trainers and racing stables and I supposed that the military powers had lost me.

When war broke out in 1939, the army wrote to tell me that vets were exempt from military service, being potentially more useful in connection with agricultural production. As I was running a veterinary practice entirely based on racing and my racing work was rapidly melting away as racing was shelved during the war, I was unemployed, so I approached the army again.

The Army hunted around and thought I might be useful to animal transport and they offered me a veterinary post connected with animal transport which was becoming urgently necessary in combating the Japanese in Burma, threatening to invade India. Animal transport sounded old fashioned, but monsoon weather, which was frequent in that combatant area, rendered mechanical transport useless except on the very few metalled roads: horses could not take the climatic conditions and animal transport meant mules.

I was given the inevitable course of twelve weeks of essential basic training in England back to drills, marching, shooting, during which my calf muscles flourished so satisfactorily that, having struggled into my riding boots with great difficulty, they had to be cut off me and thrown away. I was then posted to India by sea via South Africa. They found me a berth on the Empress of Japan, altered during the voyage to the Empress of Edinburgh, a 2nd lieutenant, as an 'officer without troops' bound for Durban. The Empress was licensed to carry 450 passengers and crew and sailed with something over 2,000, with no obvious problems. The administration was excellent and the voyage was uneventful, apart from changes in the number of ships in the convoy and its escorting naval warships, and the mystery of one man overboard, never denied or confirmed. Our course was erratic, we sailed south or north or on any other compass bearing from time to time, sometimes alone, sometimes in convoy. Those of us who enquired why were politely told that it was for 'navigational necessity': which proved successful, as the Empress reached Durban without opposition of any sort.

It took us over a month to get to Durban where, after a few days our group joined the Duchess of Bedford for a quicker leg. The convoy took nearly three months to deliver us to Bombay. The time was not wasted. Some Indian teachers on the Empress offered to teach anybody interested the Indian language of Urdu, which was the official Indian Army language and was the one most widely understood throughout India. As our group of 'officers without troops' found that time hung rather heavily, most of us joined the classes, where we learned to speak and read and write in Urdu. How the others fared, I don't know, but for me it was not only an interesting pastime because, though I was not aware of it, one of the essentials of pay and promotion for officers into the Indian Army was fluency in Urdu. We had been adequately taught and I had no difficulty in passing the necessary examinations which gave me promotion to Captain almost immediately, which was a move in the right direction. Life was full of surprises. Some of the convoy had left Durban for Singapore which had, in the meantime, fallen to the Japs. Presumably the convoy was diverted but we had no means of finding out.

Bombay

A group of about a dozen junior officers was lodged in a hostel in Bombay, enjoying life ashore and given membership of the prestigious yacht club which was friendly and luxurious. Those of us who rode were invited to hunt with the Bombay Hounds on horses provided by the Governor of Bombay. I only had one day with the hounds and was interested to meet with what were to me an unusual series of obstacles to jump: mullahs, which are water jumps and rice field boundaries (rice fields must be flooded so they must be level, and the next field may be anything from a foot to six feet higher or lower); huge sloping banks, probably involving water too as, in the rains, water takes over; and bamboo plantations. I gathered that hounds were hunting jackals though I never saw the quarry, nor the hounds very often. They went at a great pace. I contacted the Bombay Jockey Club veterinary surgeon and was invited to a race meeting, divided equally between races for thoroughbreds and those for Arabs. Altogether it was quite difficult to remember that there was a war on. I arranged for my pay to be accepted by Lloyds Bank. The Lloyds Bank manager in Swindon had said goodbye to me sitting alone in his comfortable office with the only item on his desk a large Queen Elizabeth rose bud in a vase. The manager in Bombay registered me at high speed when I reached him in the constant stream of ledger clerks who apparently ran a double entry system, each entry had to be checked and initialled personally by the manager, and everybody in the small office had a lot to say and had to say it very loud to be heard: rather like a successful cocktail party. The heat was intense and back in the main banking hall I wondered that the ink hadn't evaporated from the ink wells. Then I saw a minion going round filling up the inkpots – with clear water! This was the tropics all right! Bombay, to me, will always be hot and dry. I was only there twice, for a few days on arriving in India and for a few days on leaving. By contrast, the only other big Indian city I saw, Calcutta, was hot and wet on each of my visits and I can't imagine it in any other condition.

Before long I got used to white robed black babus cycling with their umbrellas up to shade passengers. We came across the bearer system: if there is a system. Bearers just happen. An Indian offers to help you with your luggage. You ask him who he is and he says in English 'I am your bearer, Sir.' If you ask him for references he will produce them in favourable terms, signed by a high-ranking person. They are of no importance as they can probably be purchased for a rupee or two, but bearers all seem to be honest. The person in charge of your hostel or hotel, who presumably knows your bearer, will tell you the local rate for bearers: a few rupees a week, a rupee being about five shillings. Your bearer knows where you have come from, how long you are here for and sleeps outside your door. He knows all about the locality, anticipates your requirements, deals with your laundry, does your shopping, arranges transport and is indispensable. He knows, probably before you do, what is to be your next move. For local movements, he will pack your belongings in your bedding roll and transport it for you. For major moves on your post, of which he is fully informed, he will not accompany you and he will shed no tears. When you arrive at your destination, an Indian will appear and offer to help you with your luggage.

Kashmir

I thoroughly enjoyed the company and the exercise for about three weeks when my group, now down to six or seven, was posted to an 'officers' training school', somewhere in Kashmir. We arrived in fog but, when that lifted, we had most spectacular views of conifer clad, snow-capped mountains around us. We were in the Himalayan foothills, how high I don't know but the weather was remarkable: bitterly cold and snowing every night, and it was so hot every day that the slightest breeze or traffic on the cleared roads raised dust storms.

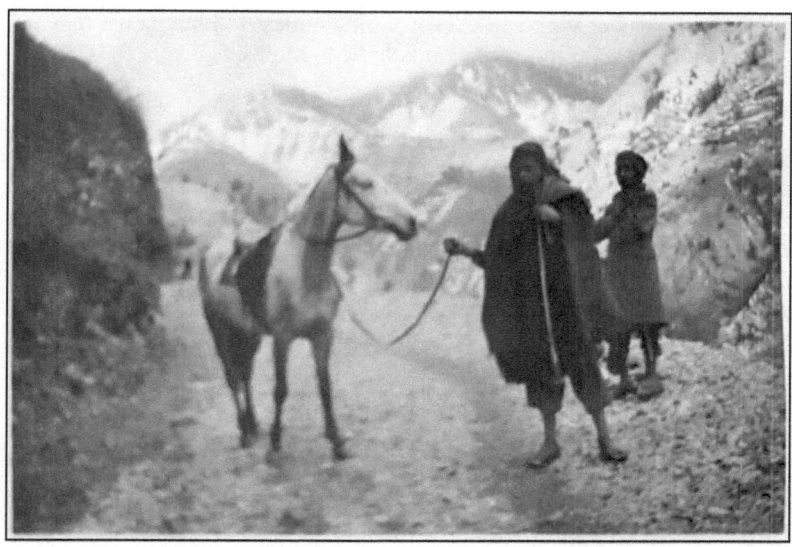

Snow-capped mountains in the Himalayan foothills

The administrative offices were quite pleasant buildings but our accommodation was under canvas. The group I was with all developed the most awful catarrhal colds and we must have created a most unfavourable impression. We stayed there three weeks, bringing the training staff up to date on modern warfare techniques. The Army in India was so solidly established in custom and use that they found the war and the impatience of all these people from England an intolerable disruption. Many unhappy days of psychological assessment followed. We none of us felt that we could justify our existence, let alone hint at our special abilities or achievements. Wherever they sent us could only be a relief. One young man with legal qualifications learned that he was to stay on the school staff, whereupon he drank himself into a fury and told the commandant in such lurid language what he could do with his school that they cancelled the invitation. Where he was posted to we never found out, but he accompanied several of us to Delhi and was so belligerently drunk that we were seriously thinking of restraining him for our and his safety when he lurched across the carriage and hit his head against a stanchion, knocking himself unconscious. We laid him on his bedding roll and locked him in an empty compartment. We kept an eye on him until he got off the train at Delhi. As so frequently happens in wartime, you meet them and lose them and wonder what happened to them.

After these gruelling interviews, I found myself posted to a Colonel Ellis who was commanding a training depot for mules at Jullundur in the Punjab. He made me a company commander and gave me a book he had written on training mules and I really felt I was in a worthwhile job at last. His requirements of me were that I could ride, speak Urdu, run a military company and like

23

mules. I could answer yes to all except 'liking mules' as I had never met any but I liked horses so I'd try to be sympathetic to mules.

Jullundur Mules

When the 1939-45 war stopped all horse racing, I was sent to India where the Japanese were invading via Burma. Frequent monsoons and no metalled roads made mechanical transport useless and mules were used by all the armies concerned. I was put in veterinary command of their breaking and training, ready for issue to Indian, British, East African and any other armies opposing the Japanese. The Japanese had wiped out the American Army, Navy and Airforce at Pearl Harbour without declaring war and proceeded to invade India via Burma.

The mule training company I was sent to command was under the direction of a Colonel Barraclough Ellis who really knew how to train mules. The mules arrived by train at Jullundur[20] in the Punjab, not far from Lahore. It seems they were purchased in South America, completely untrained: driven like a flock of sheep onto a boat, driven on arrival in India to railway trucks and unloaded from the train into the station yard at Jullundur. If you wonder how these animals were able to survive the weeks and weeks that that journey must have taken, I can only say that they all arrived in good condition. The Mule is unbelievably tough.

The mules arrived by train in batches, once a fortnight. They were untrained, not wild animals, but raised as flocks rather like sheep, used to being reasonably fenced with their dams for a year, then weaned and 'shepherded' for three years before being driven into a ship's hold and sent, still individually unhandled, to India to be trained for pack transport. The raw material that we had to work on was regularly a new group of forty or fifty unbroken, four- or five-year old mules, arriving at intervals of about three weeks.

On arrival at Jullundur the trainload was released into a yard and driven to the depot. The yard had a runway that narrowed to a one-mule wide exit. As the leading mule reached the narrowed exit, crossbars were slid into place in front of it and behind it. The single mule, penned in this way, then had a strong head collar with a rope attached slipped on and buckled. The front bars were slipped out and the mule was led or pulled to a fixed ring in the ground to which the lead rope was tied. From that moment, the mule was an individual animal, no longer one of a herd.[21]

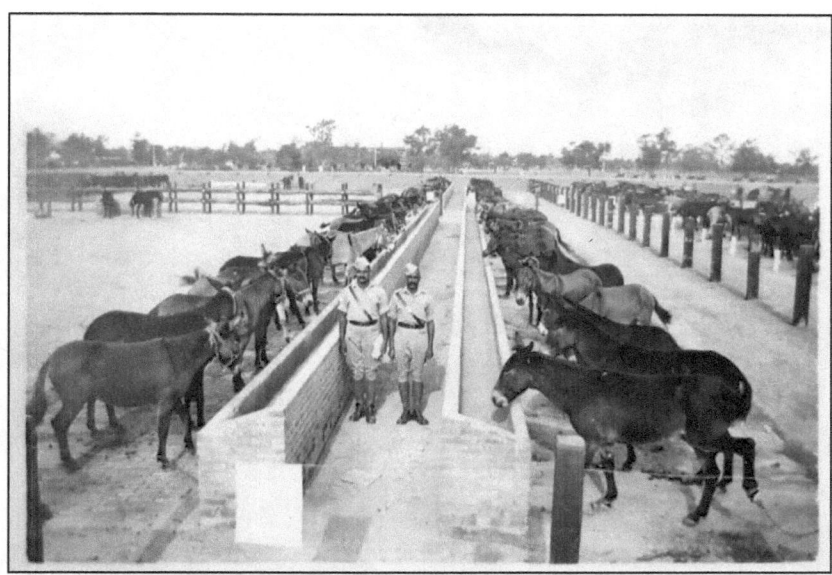

Mules at the water trough, Ambala, c.1940

Each mule was fed with hay placed conveniently near its fixed ring in the mangers and watered by being led or pulled to a water trough. The rules were strict. Any requirement of the mule had to be applied with sufficient force to overcome any resistance it could muster, so that the mule could never win. No mule was ever struck. Their intelligence was remarkable and their memories extremely good. Their first walk to the water trough was likely to be rather a struggle but, after a few visits, they knew their thirst was to be quenched and they would take the walk willingly. Twice a day green food was offered attached to a loop at the end of a foot pole and the grass was readily eaten by the mule. The groom then rubbed the mule with the end of a stick. They hated being touched, but gradually associated the touching with the attractive food.

At the end of the week, the groom who had daily shortened his hold on the stick could touch the mule by hand. At the end of two weeks he could groom the mule all over with a brush. Then leading commenced, or rather pulling. Eight men took the mule for a walk before the green stuff feed. Within a few days, habit began to creep in. The routine of walk and back to a feed could be conducted by only two men.

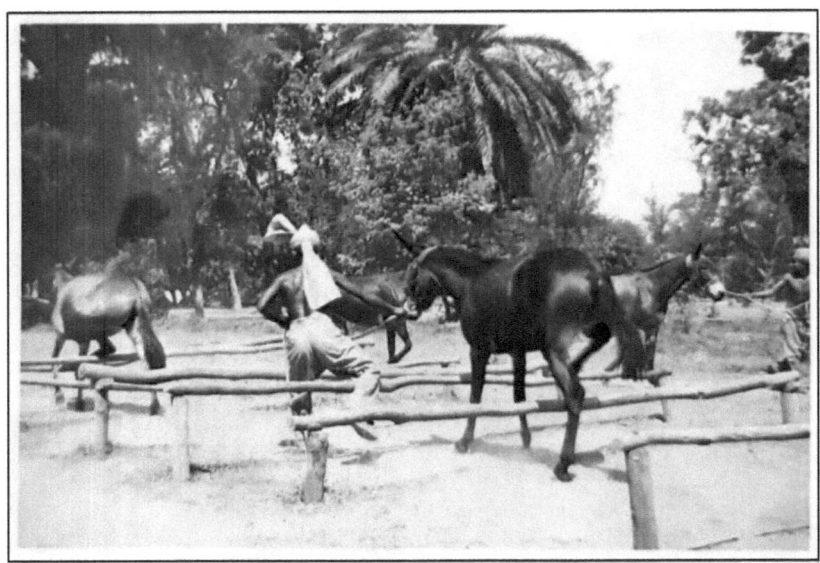

As stubborn as a mule on The Obstacle Course

A saddle was added and then a load and then The Obstacle Course was visited. Basic training depended on the observation that, as with all equine animals, they enjoyed familiar surroundings and, though always wary of anything unfamiliar, repetition without any painful content soon transferred that item to the list of familiar things. Once mules have found these unfamiliar things harmless, they accept them and are no longer frightened, so the obstacle course was designed to familiarise the mules with the whole collection of things they might find spooky in their work in town or country or on the battle field. Ingenuity was required to invent a range of items that would comprehensively include all the probable horrors of warfare which the mules should hopefully learn to be harmless, such as wooden bridges, narrow and dark trenches, motor traffic, especially motor bikes, galloping horses, flags, crowds, gunfire, dive bombing and low-flying aircraft, the closer unfamiliarity of rattling roads, harness trailing, empty cans and balloons, deep water that they learn to enjoy swimming in, and military bands especially a bagpipe band in case Scottish regiments might be encountered.

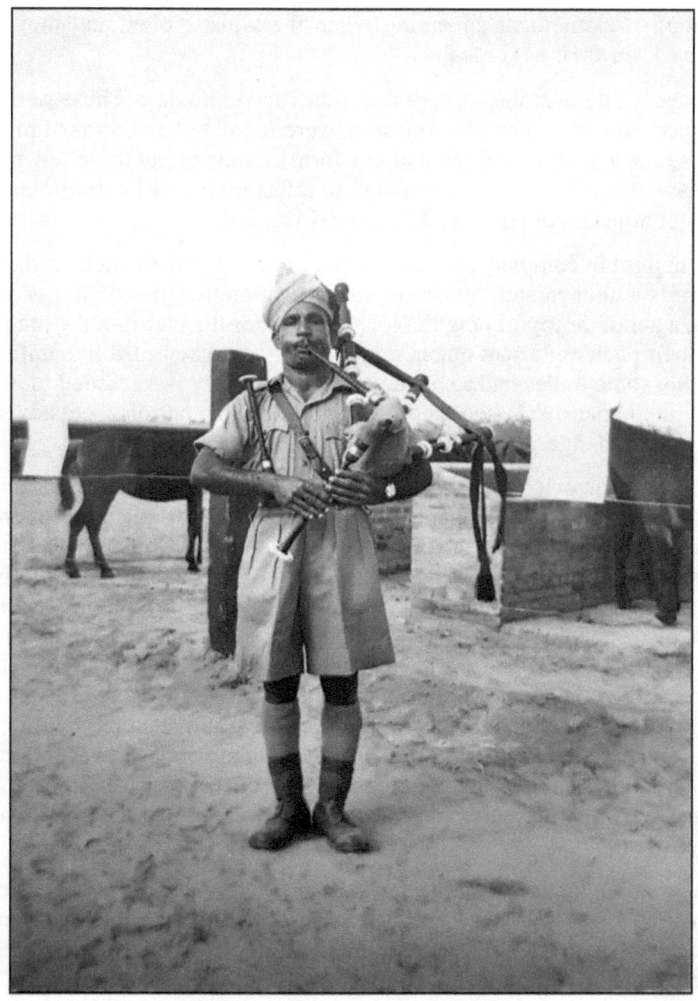

The important task of acclimatising mules to bagpipes

Compulsion might be necessary at first, eight men and a strong rope to the head collar. No mule was ever struck. If it refused to cross a rattling bridge it was dragged over, maybe on its back. Try again, this time probably on its reluctant feet. Try again. A hesitant walk. Fourth time, no pulling. So, rattling bridges don't bite after all. If there was a tasty morsel as a reward, and the exercise was repeated daily, before the end of the week one man could lead the mule over, there would be no hesitation and he might even be pulled off his feet by the mule's anxiety to get to the reward – almost like a cocky student saying "I've done bridges!". A fortnight on the course had nearly all the mules calmly facing as near all hell let loose as we could manage with their only sign of excitement appearing when the whistle blew and they could hurry back for their next meal.

I said nearly all the mules. A very few didn't accommodate. These were carefully checked and, in nearly every case, were found to have signs of previous injury. Quite a number had scars of one form or another but these few failures must have had injuries serious enough to affect their usual extraordinary capacity for adjustment and they had to be discarded.

Mules delight in company and an isolated mule is liable to check if there are any others within earshot by whinnying, which dictionaries define as 'producing a gentle or joyful neigh'. Not so joyful for the patrol in the jungle when their pack mule sent out an enquiry that could be heard five miles away. So, some mules had to be devoiced before they were issued to penetrating jungle patrols. When these were not available patrols were advised of the special danger of using single mules.

During the year or so I spend at Jullundur, my time was divided between being responsible for a company of about two hundred Indian troops and supervising batches of mules in various stages of training which involved riding for several hours each day. I had passed enough Urdu examinations to justify promotion to Captain's rank and had to attend a riding school course conducted by a sadistic martinet of a Major. I survived, but more than a few of his younger pupils ended up in hospital with ulcerated knees. I persuaded Colonel Ellis to take some action and the Major was promoted to command a camel training regiment. When my time came to move on from Jullundur, I was posted as the bullying Major's second in command! However, fate was kind. The following day that posting was cancelled and I was transferred to the Royal Army Veterinary Corps which had decided that they had a role in India after all.

While at Jullundur I was allowed to help the veterinary officer occasionally from whom I was able to pick up useful information on army veterinary requirements with special reference to mules, though there were large numbers of horses, cattle, buffaloes and camels also under his care. One night there was a stampede. Most of the animals in the station were in lines in the open and, in stampede, everything gallops in all directions until jammed into a cul-de-sac, tangled up in wire fencing or quite exhausted. The veterinary hospital was overcrowded the next day, but hardly any mules, although there were more mules than anything else in Jullundur. Major Swift was not surprised. Mules join in everything, but they are not accident prone. I found this later in Burma where mountain roads frequently have precipice sides, the army mule cart had two wheels and is pulled by two mules. The outside mule likes to look down over the edge and the inside mule jealously wants to look too. Consequently, one wheel goes over the edge and mules and cart go down the cliff side. Rescue parties were accustomed to finding one broken cart and two mules grazing alongside. Some people think mules have a sense of humour.

They certainly enjoy a stampede!

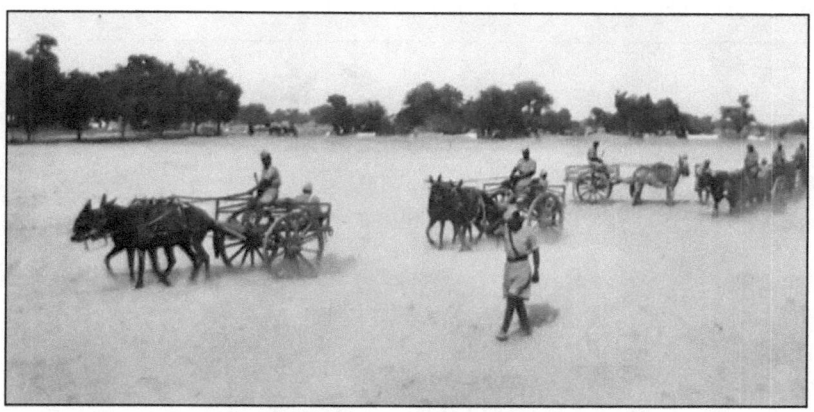

Two-wheel, two-mule carts – not a job for an inquisitive mule on a precipice

Habib Khan

One of the young Indian soldiers in my company was due for an annual fort-night's leave. He was entitled to be away for five weeks because the trip home, somewhere near the north-west frontier could take a good ten days, three days by train, seven days walking. He asked permission to take his rifle with him. I asked why. He was a Pathan from the frontier region towards Afghanistan and he said he needed the rifle because he had an urge, or per-haps a moral responsibility to level a score. There was a current feud at home and he would be required to avenge his uncle's death. Not being informed about tribal customs, I consulted Colonel Ellis who said "ABSOLUTELY NOT!", it was out of the question, so Habib went off unarmed. He came back two months later and was automatically brought before me on a charge of being two or three weeks absent without leave. He regretted the delay but he had had difficulty in finding a rifle to settle the feud problems. He bore no resentment and I gathered that he had enjoyed his leave as he had eventually been able to borrow a gun!

He accepted three weeks in the cells as inevitable and, on his release he asked, as my groom batman had been promoted, if he could have the job. I agreed. He was a champion wrestler and a good horseman and he looked after me well. Like most Orientals prestige was important to him. Out riding one day, his horse came past me with an empty saddle. I caught it up and took it back to him and we rode on, but he was very subdued and remained so for a day or two. I was wondering if I should enquire what was amiss, but we were crossing some rice fields in an irrigated area, the next field being three feet above the one we were in. My horse at a canter never rose at all, hit the bank chest high and shot me face first into the higher field. Habib collected my horse and happily dug me out of the mud. Whatever loss of face he had been harbouring was apparently eliminated by my relapse and I had no further need to complain about his lack of cheerfulness.

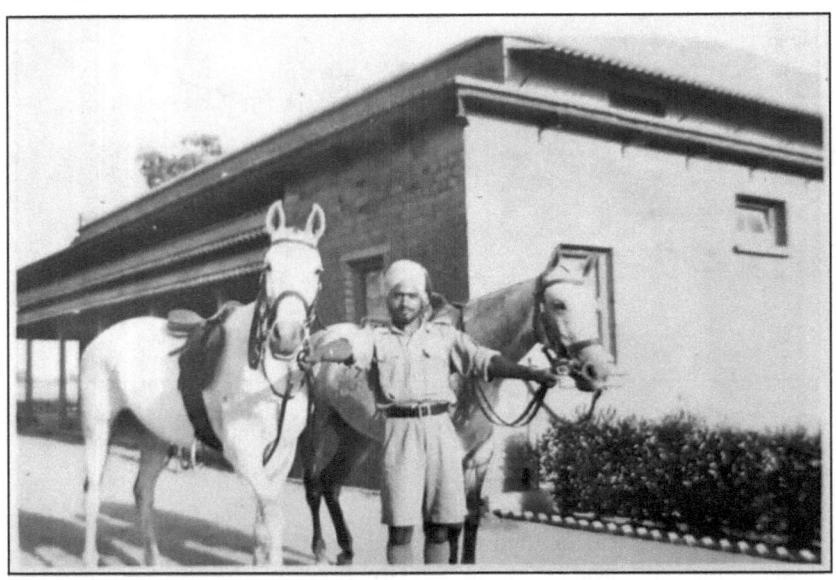

Photo of an Indian solider from Alistair's company, possibly Habib Khan

I asked him if he would train me to be a farrier and he put me through the full course in farriery as the Indian soldiers were trained. He just had me for half an hour or so in the lunch hour for a month or more. He produced a piece of iron rod from which I had to cut off the length I wanted to make a shoe, and then put in the furnace, turn the blast to get the iron red hot, then hammer it into the shape of a shoe with a suitable thickness and so on. I had to make the toe clip and bend it into the right shape and then turn the ends down to make the heels. Then he commandeered the local mule cart that did a tour each night and emptied the "drops" from the various lavatories. Over several weeks, I would take one of the shoes off under his instruction and made a suitable shoe to fit this mule. I'd done quite a bit of removing shoes but I'd just ripped them off, he showed me the farriery way of taking a shoe off properly and then preparing the foot and adjusting the shoe. Then I actually nailed on the shoe, which is the trickiest bit because if you get a nail too deep it lames the animal with a nasty kind of lameness which takes a long time to develop. The mule was then trotted up on the hard road and it wasn't lame. Then to my horror he took the shoe off and put it on again, just to make a job of it. I was issued with a certificate to the effect that I had passed the farriery exam satisfactorily, which he said he hadn't had to stretch his conscience very far to issue. I was then officially listed as having passed the elementary examination for farriers to the Indian Army Standard.

Camels

There was a camel training unit not far from the mule training location at Jullundur and there was some question as to whether I should be transferred to that outfit, but nothing came of it. As far as I could find out, the camels didn't need training. They joined the army with their owners: one man and two camels, rather like the British yeomanry, when young farmers joined up with their own horses.

The Indian camels are mostly situated in the Himalayan foothills, the plains being unsuitable for them in the monsoon weather owing to the prevalence of the disease Surra, a kind of malaria of camels, horses and mules, transmitted by biting flies. While I was in the Punjab, on the plain, a number of civilian-owned camels were working for the Army. Their home was in the hills six hundred miles away. They moved in the Spring from the hills to the plain, travelling twenty miles a night for thirty nights. There they worked for six months, each day consisting of transport work from midnight until 8am at the coolest part of the day. They then grazed on camel thorn for 8 hours until 4 o'clock and rested in camp to digest their food or ruminate until work started again at 12. With the hot weather tailing off and the onset of the rains, the whole company marched back home, taking a further month to catch up with their family affairs and the local gossip, and for a four-month respite.

There are no wild camels. The camel people breed and rear their animals in the home almost – because of teething problems. The process in camels of replacing milk teeth with the adult set is so fraught with sore gums that they are not able to eat heartily enough to cope with the demands of both growth and work. So, they are idle about the homestead and there is plenty of time to accustom them to saddles and loads and discipline.

Working with camels and their owners took one back to a centuries old way of life. One young British officer, attached to a camel transport unit, told me his men enjoyed nothing better than him reading to them selected portions of the Old Testament in Urdu. I can think of no setting so romantic as being in the company of a camel caravan on the sandy roads with no light but the brilliant stars and no sound except the beautiful singing voices of the young men leading the camels.

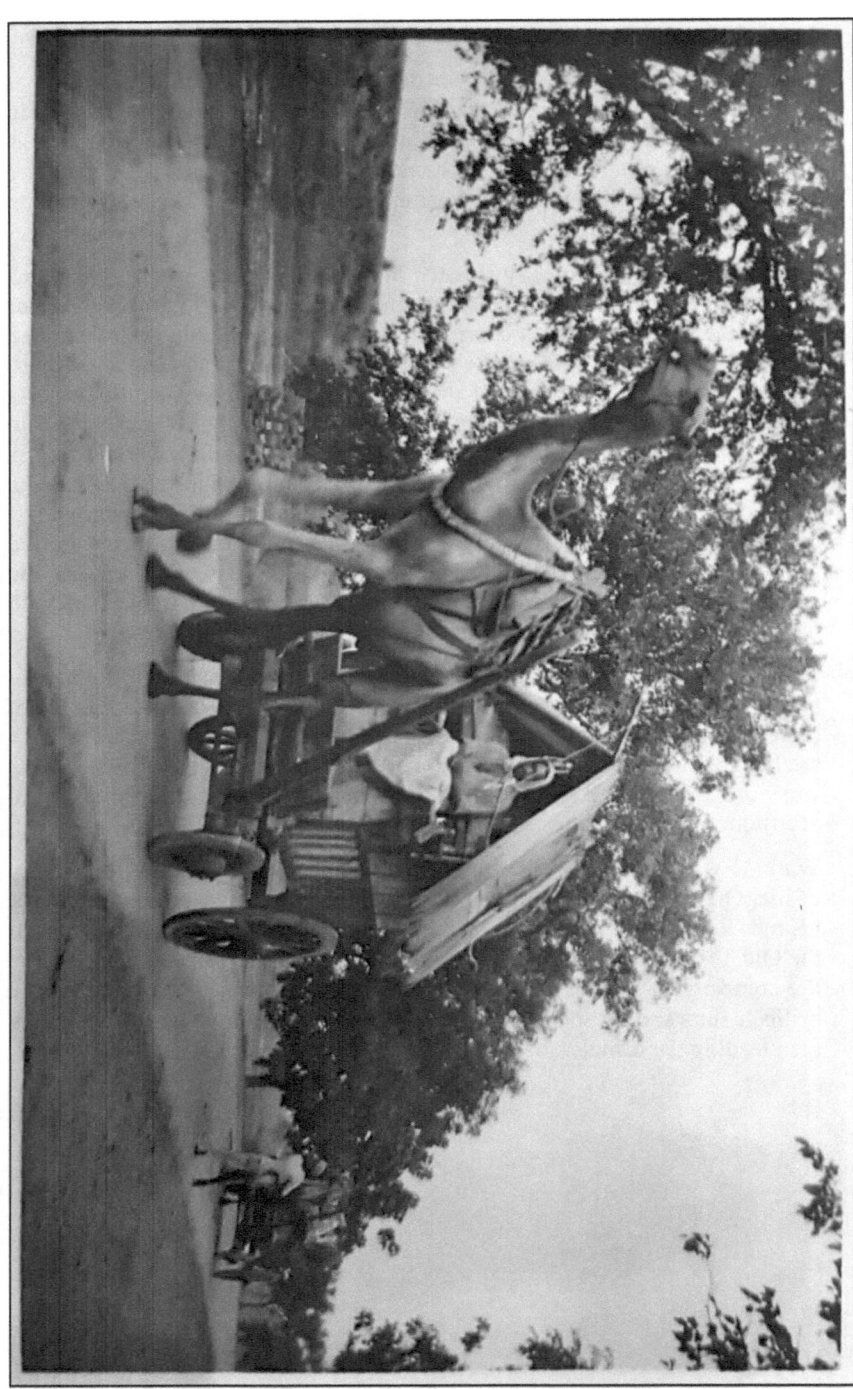

It is easier for a camel to go through the eye of a needle than for it to pull this contraption

Private Veterinary Practice in India

I only had one day of private veterinary practice in India. I was at the Indian Army Veterinary Corps headquarters at Ambala in the Punjab assembling a mobile veterinary hospital of thirty dressers, one Indian veterinary surgeon, five ambulance trucks and myself, to go eventually to the Arakan area of south Burma, where the Japanese, who had captured Rangoon, were attempting to penetrate to the north. Transport for the armies involved was a severe problem as monsoon conditions, over several months twice a year, immobilised motorised vehicles, thrusting their work on to pack transport by mules, hundreds of which my mobile veterinary hospital was intended to care for when necessary.

One day, Colonel Barnett, in command of the Ambala veterinary centre, told me that the Maharajah of Sirmoor State[22] had bought ten riding horses, on condition that they were found to be 'sound' by a British veterinary surgeon; and the Colonel said that, if I cared to respond to this rather unusual request, I could have a day's leave for the purpose.

I chose my day and Sirmoor state said they would arrange transport from the railway station at Kissangar, thirty miles by rail from Ambala, which they did most efficiently. My bearer woke me up at 4 o'clock and I took a taxi (a tonga drawn by two trotting bullocks) to Ambala station, catching my train at 5 a.m. A twenty seater bus was waiting for me at Kissangar. This took me fifteen miles towards the foothills of a village where an annual buffalo market was in full swing. (Buffalo supply the small Indian farmer's horsepower.)

As metalled roads went no further, the bus driver handed me over to a Sirmoor groom who was waiting with two saddled horses to take me nine miles to the Sirmoor State border. We forded two deep streams and were finally faced by quite a deep river, about fifty yards wide, which was not suitable for the horses to cross. While I was wondering whether to wade or swim, I was picked up by a muscular Indian who carried me over with no problems, until he slipped just before reaching the far bank and I was well and truly ducked. I had spare clothes so tightly packed in a haversack that they were quite dry when, after another bus had run me five miles uphill through lovely jungle country, we arrived at Sirmoor and I was able to change into dry clothes and enjoy a late breakfast.

Sirmoor is a small town, built up on three hills around a level green of five or six acres. The Maharajah was in a Calcutta hospital for some treatment so I was greeted by his prime minister and the usual set in such principalities of high ranking and English-speaking officials, but I finally found my way to the stables and the Indian veterinary surgeon, who welcomed me for sharing his responsibilities. I rode each of the animals; five ride and drive horses and five polo ponies; in pouring rain on the central area of level common, watched by several hundred men, women and children; most of Sirmoor's population,

I imagine.

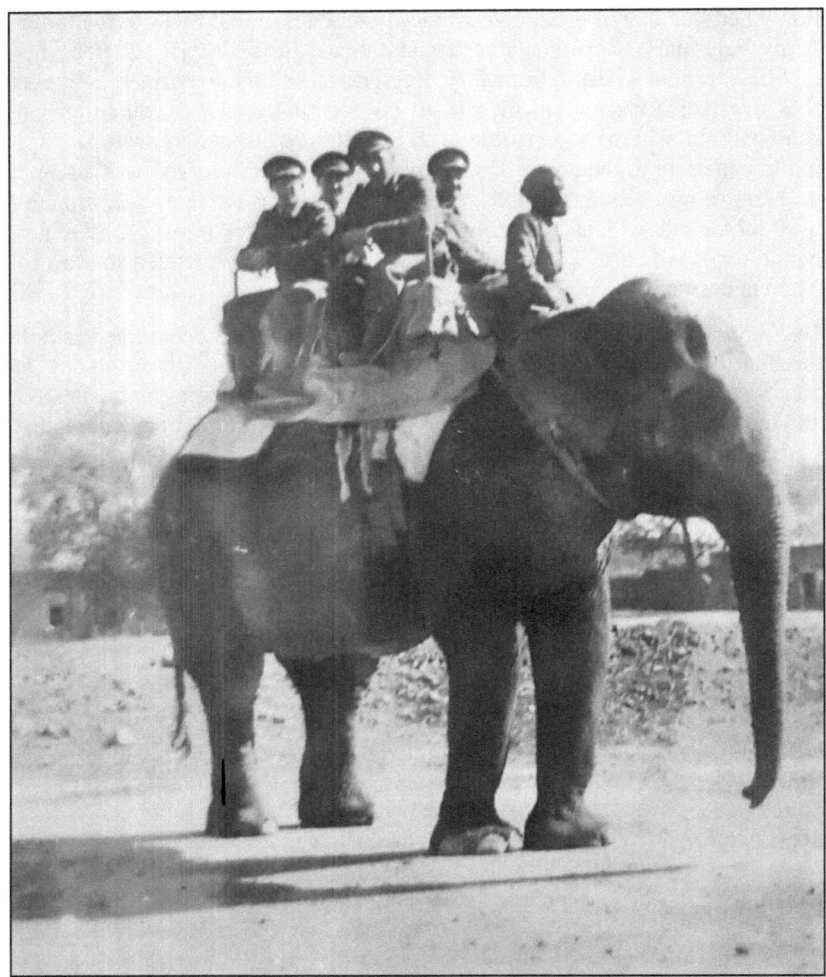

Riding the Maharajah of Sirmur's elephant

To my relief, I found nothing seriously amiss with any of the animals. I did the necessary paperwork and, after lunch, had each of the animals trotted out, and still found them to be adequately in order. I settled up with the financial secretary and then found that I was expected to stay the night. I declined, which they assumed was just politeness on my part, but I finally convinced them that I was leaving and they produced the bus to take me down to the river. The horse dealer's representative, who had brought the horses from Calcutta, asked if he could join me as he too, wanted to get back to the railway station. I was glad to have his company then, and even more so later. He was a Sikh and, as most Sikhs seem to be, he was large and strong. The river was wider and deeper than it had been earlier in the day, so the bus could not cross. No problem! He picked me up and carried me over without missing his footing: and we set off for the nine mile walk to the buffalo market village where the hard roads began.

The weather had changed to a beautiful moonlight night, and for mile after mile, the sides of the path were lined with myriads of fireflies, which my Sikh companion called Titana. We had no language problem. He had enough English and I had enough Urdu for us to get along very well together. I would have imagined that a nine mile walk at night in the approaches to the Himalayas could be eerie, lonely and hilly. Having done it that morning on horseback I knew it would be level. The southern edge of the Himalayas is like that. The hills started at the Sirmoor river border. The north bank rises, the south bank is flat.

We walked on the level, but by no means alone. We met dozens of people taking advantage of the cool, fine night to get on with furniture moving and other major activities that would not have been easy in the rain and heat of the previous day. Wildlife was plentiful too, and extremely noisy: bats, owls, jackals and small packs of wild (ownerless mongrel) dogs: with all, except the bats, loudly voicing their presence, with not the slightest hint of the "stealth-by-night" that I would have expected.

A minor item of surprise was to see milestones with consecutive numbers from the Sirmoor river. My Sikh companion sat me down by milestone nine and went into the village, telling me that he would arrange transport to the railway station if I would pay for it. I readily agreed. Time went by, but I was too tired to worry and eventually he came back with the bus and the driver I had used the previous morning. For an amount equivalent to fifteen shillings, we were driven to Kissangar, arriving there as a train for Ambala drew into the station at 2 o'clock in the morning. Whether that was an example of extreme efficiency or sheer luck I shall never know. I was back in my bed almost exactly twenty-four hours after leaving it. I spent the next day supervising students taking a written examination; an ideal occupation requiring no exertion and giving me time to consider how very thoroughly the British Empire in India had been co-ordinated, and to be rather surprised to have found that nobody in Sirmoor seemed to know that there was a war on.

Bihar and Burma

I joined the 5th Indian Division which was assembling in Bihar preparatory to moving into Burma. I found my veterinary hospital was alongside a medical hospital, commanded by a Colonel Stephenson who was a veterinary surgeon as well as being a doctor and he kindly invited me to join his mess which was friendly of him as I was entirely staffed by Indians which meant I had to mess alone. As we were moving to Burma where monsoons are frequent, making mechanical transport impossible, Colonel Stephenson had eight officer's chargers (riding horses) for his doctors to get about. He asked me to look after the horses which suited me as I had none on my strength. We then found that the division was doubling; to be made into two divisions so that the Colonel was issued with sixteen horses, all at my disposal. I ran a riding school for his officers and conducted my duties of visiting units with mules and horses, escorted by a dozen or so of my veterinary corps dressers, which caused amusement when I arrived and was found to be a mere Captain.

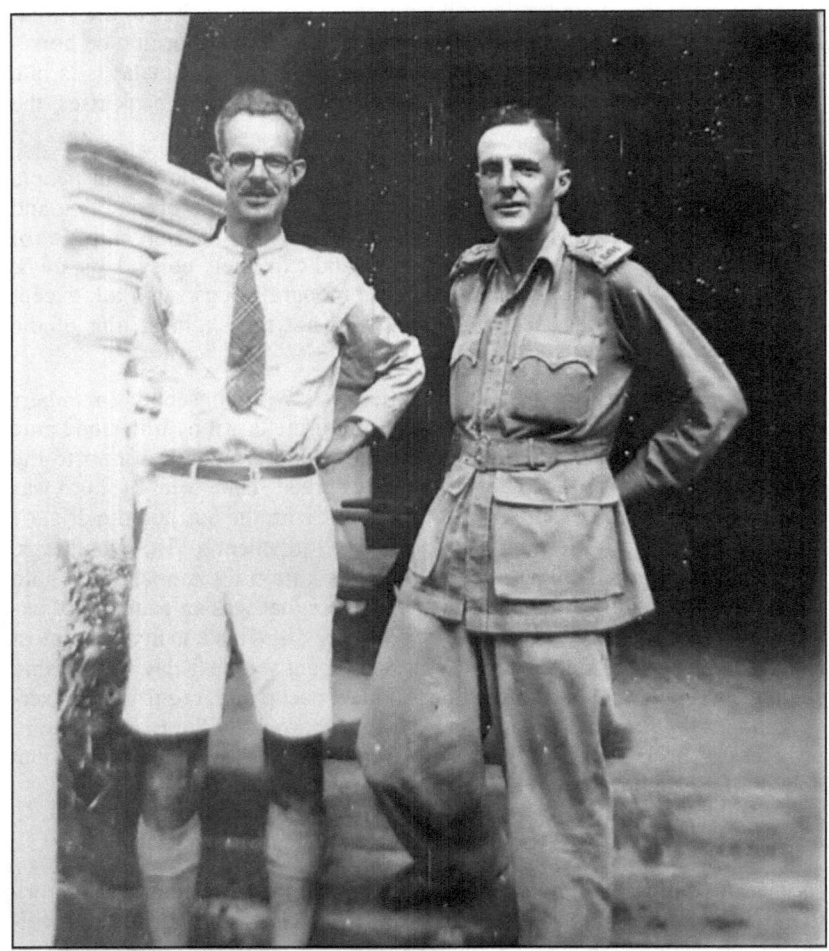

Dr Neil Fraser (1900-1969), reunited in India with his brother Alistair

At that time, I had a letter from my father telling me that my doctor brother, Neil was in some trouble in China, where the Japanese were advancing down the coast where Neil was, and that he had had to move inland and from one town to another. My father gave me Neil's latest address. I was mentioning this to American Air Force pilots I met in Ranchi and they said they were supplying the Chinese forces from India and coming back empty so, if Neil went to an USA aerodrome in China, they'd fly him out. So, I wrote an air letter to Neil in China, assuming that it would not reach him through the Japanese lines and forgot about it but, six weeks later, he walked into my hospital. The USA had flown him to Calcutta and he went to Army HQ and demanded to know where I was. We had a party and he went off to Australia to join his wife and family who had evacuated from China six months earlier.

During the invasion, the Japanese over-ran the big veterinary hospital which I had been building up. Luckily for me, I had been recalled to deal with a Swine Fever outbreak in Agra as the only veterinary surgeon east of Suez known to have written up that disease – but that was work done in 1926 with my uncle, and this was 1944! Knowledge of Swine Fever, however limited and out of date, had saved my life.

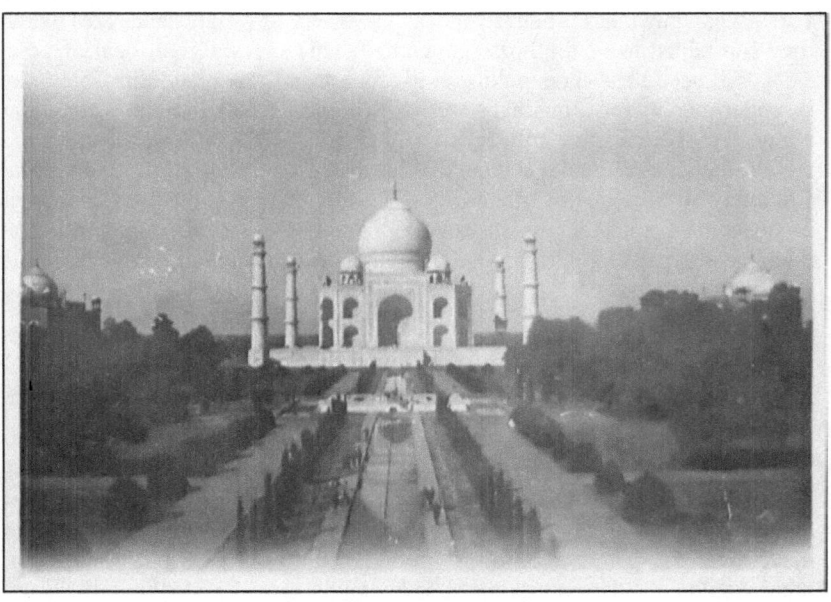

Alistair's photo of the Taj Mahal in Agra, he was fortuitously recalled here during the Japanese invasion of Burma

Part 3 – Veterinarian at Work

Farriery

Farriers are blacksmiths who shoe horses. Their work has two facets: making the shoes and nailing them onto a horse's hoof. Working horses need shoes whether they are at work on hard or soft surfaces. The friction of hard or rough going wears out or chips off the hoof horn: wet going softens the horn so that the feet break and bruise easily. The iron shoe nailed to the hoof protects the foot from wear. The horny rim of the hoof grows like a finger nail. In the wild this growth is enough to compensate for the wear and tear of the horse's natural activities. In shod horses the horn continues to grow, lengthening the foot which, if allowed to persist, alters the horse's stride and balance and may give rise to strains and injuries: so shoes have to be taken off every month or so, to allow the hoof growth to be trimmed. A new shoe is then attached or, if the old one is not too worn, that one is re-applied.

Farriers are trained to make shoes and to fit them to a particular horse when they have suitably prepared each foot for the shoe to be applied. Apprentices spend three years in practical and theoretical work at college and with a master and must pass a series of examinations to qualify and become registered as farriers. Horse shoeing by unregistered persons is against the law.

Farriers can buy mass produced shoes in a variety of weights and sizes which they can adjust to fit the horse concerned. This saves a great deal of time. They still need their shoe making skills for special cases, and this point may be underlined by recalling that a very critical old farrier examiner's comment about any of his expert colleagues was always "Oh yes. He's a very good farrier, but he can't make a shoe!". With the co-operation of the Worshipful Company of Farriers, one of the City of London Livery companies, a number of agricultural societies run shoe-making and horse-shoeing competitions at their shows, the competitions leading to the election annually of a Champion Farrier of England.

Every now and again some ingenious person, exasperated by the nuisance of shoeing, invents a shoe that doesn't need to be nailed using some strap or glue, but shoes have been nailed on for about 2,500 years and that still seems to be essential.

Veterinary surgeons are responsible for all types of disease and injury and, when a horse's foot is involved, they often find that they need the assistance and co-operation of a farrier. Most veterinary surgeons can take a shoe off to make a careful examination of an injured or diseased foot, but very few of them would consider putting the shoe back on again. This is the farrier's department and, if one is available, it is sensible to have him take the shoe off and co-operate in any remedial shoeing that may be required, as it is he who will be doing the mechanical adjustments and re-applying the shoe.

There are always borderline cases as to the divisional responsibility but in foot cases the veterinary surgeon and the farrier can usually work amicably together, bearing in mind their responsibility to the horse and to the owner who is paying them both to get his horse back to work as soon as possible.

As a youngster still at college, I was lucky to be temporarily in charge of a veterinary practice in Liverpool and to find myself the boss for a month of a three-fired forge: that meant three anvils and six men, three of them being firemen (making the shoes) and three strikers (who nailed them on). My overseeing really only meant that I paid the wages. The forge belonged to a veterinary surgeon who had shoeing contracts with a number of transport companies. I was lucky to have the opportunity of seeing farriers in action at close quarters and luckier perhaps that no serious veterinary problems on feet arose: though I would have been permitted to call in more experienced veterinary advice if necessary. Foot abscesses were frequent in horses whose shoes had been poorly nailed. Once the abscess burst, fluid would spurt out in a spectacular jet. As an antiseptic, a little turpentine poured onto iodine crystals laid in the cavity then ignited itself with a sudden cloud of blue smoke and the horse, freed of pain, would start to eat again.

Colonel Miller

Colonel Miller (now Sir John[23]), the crown equerry, was a man of very direct action. A typical example was when he was summoned to Windsor Castle he said to the soldier who was driving his jeep, 'go straight up to the castle.' The driver said 'I can't, sir. It's a one-way street.' Colonel Miller pushed him out of the vehicle and drove himself straight there.

He was told one evening that a horse at the London Mews had cut itself and that the head groom couldn't stop the bleeding. He rang my surgery at Wokingham and was told that I was at a meeting in London but that another veterinary surgeon was available. He demanded to know where I was and 'phoned an urgent message for my attention. This was 10 o'clock at night and, luckily, the meeting was not over. I went to the Mews, but I had no veterinary equipment. I needed a pair of artery forceps. Mine were 20 miles away. I managed to borrow a pair from the casualty officer at a London hospital and all was well. Soon after I got home, Colonel Miller rang through to say he had had a report from Showell, the head groom, that the blood was staunched.

On another occasion, he found my 'phone was out of order. He rang the Wokingham police to come round and tell me to ring him back immediately. He was at a palace dinner and the Queen had heard that a case of African horse sickness had been reported in England. 'Was it true?' By a stroke of luck, I had been talking to veterinary people at the Ministry of Agriculture earlier that day and I was able to tell Colonel Miller that the nearest case was in Spain, so Her Majesty was able to enjoy her meal with, I hope, some peace of mind.

Before horses were routinely vaccinated against influenza, which began in the 1950s, 'flu epidemics were a nuisance. A Windsor horse was transferred to London on a Friday. It began to cough on Saturday, obviously had 'flu on Sunday and, by the end of the next week, most of the thirty horses in the London Mews were coughing and sneezing with a high temperature, and so no horses were available. He got on the 'phone to the Life Guards to borrow six horses. They regretted that all their horses had 'flu. This presented a diplomatic incident. Protocol required carriages and escort according to rank. I imagined that there was nothing I could do about it but apparently there was. Diplomatic etiquette was not to be flouted lightly. Somebody must accept the blame. I was responsible for the horses' health and they were all sick. Was this to be 'Off with his head!'? I was instructed to put in writing for the information of all at the Court that it was on my advice that this unfortunate gaffe had to be perpetrated. In the event, the German party was transported in Rolls Royces and Daimler cars instead of in carriages which, except in the finest weather, when they could have the hoods folded away, always smelled fusty and dusty. I didn't have to fight a duel with the German veterinary attaché.

The Royal Farriers

I found my farriery training in India very useful when I was working with the Queen's Horses and got on well with the Royal farriers. They knew their jobs a damn sight better than I did, but I was able to help them with the difficult bits. I don't mean the difficult farriery but their contact training and that sort of thing. I was always friendly with the farriers.

I was always impressed by the genuine devotion to duty of all the people in Royal Service. Two, possibly rather trivial incidents come to mind. During the King's Troop Royal Artillery galloping display at the Royal Windsor Horse Show, one of the young troopers, changing his position as a flag marker, tripped on a tent peg, fell onto the next one and was completely winded. His colleague, running past, paused to see what he could do, and the prostrate boy managed to gasp out 'Take my lance' (the master flag) 'and tell Tom'. He recovered in a couple of minutes but he'd done his best to keep the show on the road.

Another incident affected one of the London Mews farriers whose duty it was to go on the day The Queen was opening the new session of Parliament, to Parliament Square, to be available in case any of the horses had any trouble such as a loose shoe. What with the Life Guards, the Police horses and the Queen's carriage procession, there were hundreds of horses in the Parliament Square area. Colonel Miller also fixed up to have me around in case of any problems. So, I was at Buckingham Palace Mews and on call if necessary. If a horse were to go lame, they wanted a veterinary surgeon to authorise its withdrawal.

The farrier had everything ready at the Mews. He was to walk to his post, the best way to get there with the congested traffic, and it would take him a quarter of an hour. Just as he was leaving one of the mounted police pulled into the Mews to have a loose shoe clinched up. That only took a few minutes, but it made him a little late. However, he got to his nook in Parliament Square just as the first horses were arriving and very relieved to have made it, checked that he had all he required and found that he had left his bag of tools at the Mews. For two hours and a half he stood there contemplating his position. No calls were made for his services and nobody knew of his default.

I was at the Mews the next day and he asked me if I'd mind coming to his flat above the stables. His wife was out at work and he made me a cup of coffee and told me all about his experience the day before. He hadn't dared tell anybody, not even his wife, and he hadn't slept all night. Some people might have exulted that they had got away with it or thanked their lucky stars that they hadn't been found out, but his worry was partly that he hadn't done his duty and, during his vigil, he must have wondered what dire punishment Colonel Miller would have thought up for him if he found out. He certainly punished himself for his gross carelessness. I was sorry for him and glad that he was able to get it off his chest. What a subject for his nightmares! Perhaps there's some comfort that the worse the nightmare the greater the relief when you wake up.

He was a very nice chap, he was a Scot and he played the bagpipes. The Queen used him when she had any Scottish guests at her party to walk up and down outside the dining room. He'd been playing a few Scottish tunes and when Olive and I went to one of the garden parties at Buckingham Palace, he was there in a red coat taking invitation cards and checking that you were who you were supposed to be. And then a year or so later Olive and I went to another garden party and this farrier was there at the Garden Party as a guest with his wife, and I thought that was really something.

The whole set-up of Royalty is remarkably run, the Royal Family get a lot of good marks from me for the way they run the show. It's not the Queen who does everything, it's the Organisation, but the Queen can manipulate the Organisation because they know she would like this or that kind of thing.

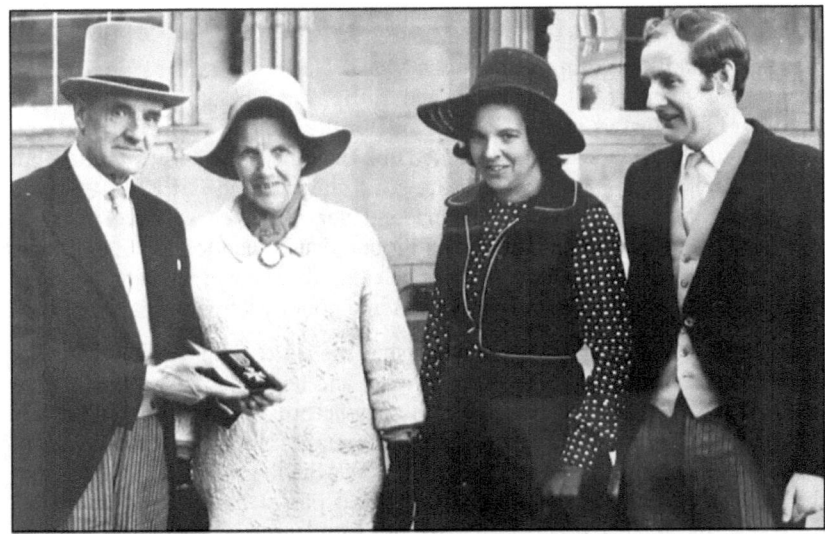

Alistair, Olive, and children Katharine and Duncan, at Buckingham Palace on the occasion of receiving the award of Lieutenant of the Royal Victorian Order, 1973

The Workshipful Company of Farriers

While I was in London doing quite a lot of work at Buckingham Palace, somebody said it would be to my advantage to join the Worshipful Company of Farriers which I arranged to do and I had to attend a meeting of the Farriery Committee. I don't think I had to pass any examination but there was a committee that interviewed me for my suitability to become a Member. I told them about my qualification and I had particulars of the standard, but I hadn't got the certificate because the hospital I had in Burma was over-run by Japs when I was away inspecting for swine fever. and the Japs had taken my certificate amongst other belongings. It was all rather a tongue in cheek interview. I said that I had passed an examination in Farriery and quoted the examinations that I'd passed. The Queen's Horse Controller, Colonel Miller was on the committee and he wondered if I might be interested to know that the Indian Army had since reviewed farriery standards and that Grade III was considered to be so elementary that it had been discontinued!.I replied that of course that would have made my certificate of even more antiquarian value. They took a vote on whether I was to join or not, and he opposed my application to join the Worshipful Company. However, as most of them had never heard of me before and I was polite to them, they outvoted Colonel Miller and I became a member of the Worshipful Company of Farriers.

I could attend their dinners in London and that kind of thing, a fiver to go to dinner and if you took a guest it was seven pounds ten for a guest. Just recently I had a circular inviting me to attend one of their annual or biennial gatherings. If I accepted the invitation to come, the ticket would cost fifty pounds and if I was to have a guest that would be sixty-five pounds. Isn't inflation extraordinary, just to have a four-course meal and couple of drinks? It is inflammation. When I finished work, I was charging Americans a thousand dollars a day plus expenses.

The Horse that wouldn't be Shod

On one occasion the farriers at the Buckingham Palace Mews asked me to give a tranquilliser to one of the carriage horses that refused to be shod. The gelding, Cambridge, weighed nearly a ton and resisted all their attempts to lift his feet from the ground. I carefully calculated the intravenous dose for a ton of sixteen-year-old horseflesh but some veterinary surgeons miscalculate and some horses are hypersensitive. Anyway, Cambridge, instead of becoming amenable, collapsed unconscious, draped over an anvil. The farriers, helped by other staff who had curiously gathered round, levered the body off the anvil onto a ten-foot-square mattress (The Royal Mews are fully equipped). The farriers then asked me what they should do. They seemed a little surprised when I said 'carry on shoeing'. I might have been amused to watch their contortions as they shod the horse lying on its side, but my thoughts were fully engaged in considering antidotes and mortality but, to my relief, just as shoeing was completed, Cambridge raised his head, adjusted his legs and got up. After a few minutes, to allow the horse to recover his wits, a groom trotted him down the yard and back again showing, to the farriers' relief, that none of their shoeing nails, which have a very narrow margin of accuracy, were pressing on sensitive tissues. A conscious horse gives a nervous reaction (as we would say 'ouch') if a nail is too tight and the farrier then realigns it. This was the first unconscious horse they had shod and they had been aware that there would be no warnings to guide their nails.

The story doesn't end there. What about subsequent shoeings? Cambridge submitted to the next shoeing session without any complaint which I found most interesting because, in the great days of the horse, when horses were almost the only source of power and transport, the specialists in mastering unruly horses were agreed that one of the greatest helps in curing stubbornness was to cast the horse onto the ground, which they would do, not by intravenous injection, but by ropes and hobbles. Perhaps my overdose was justified.

The Horse that Fainted

Another carriage horse, Sedan, caused me to receive a reprimand for my advice that might, in times past, have suddenly terminated my career. Sedan had fainted in his stall. In horses, that usually means a brain problem but this case seemed to be due to erratic heart action. The case history was that fainting in the stable had occurred several times during recent months and so Sedan was not being used on important occasions, although he was one of the horses that usually drew the Queen's carriage at Ascot. I advised the Crown Equerry that such a case might be the cause of a serious accident and that, for safety, the horse should be shot. This advice was duly reported to Her Majesty who, so I was told, replied that she was in favour of the shooting but that it was not the horse but the vet who should be destroyed. Shades of 'Off with his head' again.

The Queen's suggestion had the desired effect. Equine heart specialists were called in to make electro-cardio-graphic investigations which showed that the heart as an organ was sound, but that the nervous controls were amiss. Medicines were prescribed and Sedan was put on a programme of graded exercise. A year later he took part in a minor marathon drive from London to Windsor Mews to check his heart as well as other horses. On their arrival, Sedan's heart was just as good as any of the others, and he continued to appear in his usual role on ceremonial occasions until he retired at the age of twenty-four. I still have my head...

Thoroughbred Horses at Sea

In 1960 at one of the horse sales regularly held at Newmarket, one of the dealers told me that his firm had bought ten young horses for a trainer in Singapore. He had arranged transport with a shipping firm and everything was in hand for transport from London but, because of an outbreak of African Horse Sickness in various countries around the Mediterranean, ships carrying horses through the area must be vaccinated against that disease. However, because vaccination is a tedious affair, it was not thought necessary for small numbers of horses if they were 'adequately supervised'. Somewhat surprisingly, a veterinary surgeon on board would suffice and, as none of my colleagues showed any interest, I appointed myself as fly-repellent-in-chief.

The Ben Armin was a small cargo and passenger steamer sailing regularly to eastern ports and she was due to leave on a Friday, so I went to London on the Wednesday and found her berthed at Tilbury. Captain McNab, a gruff Aberdonian, was a man of few words. He had already completed his quota of eight passengers, so he signed me on as a member of his crew; and I would be accommodated in the ship's hospital: a small and most unattractive cabin. At best, he appeared to look upon me as a damned nuisance.

The next day two assistant trainers arrived with the horses, to care for them during the voyage. An assistant trainer leads a busy life. He usually looks after two horses in the trainer's string, attending to their grooming, feeding and exercise; jobs which fill up an eight-hour day for the other stable lads; but the assistant trainer must also find time to familiarise himself with the very complex office work which has to do with each horse's requirements and accompany the trainer to any race meeting where he has an entry. An assistant trainer needs limitless ambition to support his commitments.

These two young men, Eric and Maurice, had all the desirable qualities. They summed up Mr McNab as a bully and they told me that, if I would keep the Captain off their backs, they would look after the horses: which they did so well that, when we unloaded the horses in Singapore, they were in better condition than they had been when we left Tilbury. My job, apart from supervision, which proved unnecessary, was to keep African horse sickness at bay. One mosquito was repelled at Port Said, another at Aden, but in general, it was not flying weather.

The loading arrangements were very impressive. Each horse arrived by lorry, in a horse box that could be lifted by a crane onto the ship's high foredeck, where the boxes were lined up, five to port and five to starboard, leaving a good wedge of deck area between, to which each box had a door for access to the animal, for care and attention. In its box, each horse had just enough room to get up or lie down easily, and they could manage to turn round though they seldom did.

The efficiency of the whole process was so remarkable that I wrote that evening to the horse-dealing firm, who were employing me, to tell them how impressed I was by their organisation.

The next day, Friday, the eight passengers joined the ship and we set sail, the day being fully occupied finding our way about the ship and sorting out who were passengers, who were officers and who were crew: there were twenty-two in the crew, half British and half Chinese.

On the second day out, the Captain sent for me to say that he was moving me to the pilot's cabin, now that it was vacated. It was luxurious after the hospital bed. He also asked me to sit at his table and to join him and his officers at their conferences half an hour before lunch and again before supper, where I was surprised to be treated with some deference and gin. I couldn't account for the sea change. Perhaps McNab was only happy at sea, provided he won his evening Scrabble session.

The voyage was uneventful until, at 6 o'clock one morning, firecrackers were exploding all over the place. I never found out if it was geography indicating that we had 'crossed the line' or a calendar event: Chinese New Years seem to crop up at less than twelve-month intervals. Whatever the crackers were for, they upset the horses, which were kicking their box walls; which were not all that solid. I got hold of the first officer to restore order: and the Captain pronounced that the celebration might take place from 6 p.m. which seemed acceptable. At 5 o'clock, I gave each of the horses an injection of Acetylprom-azine. The cracker fusillade began again and hose pipes were laid out as a fire precaution. The Chinese crew ordered to stow the pipes away, turned the water on and hosed down the British, cheered on by the passengers who were enjoying the fracas until, they – and everybody else – were all thoroughly soaked, except for the two horsemen and me. We stood guard at the access to the horse deck, and the riot, which I gathered ran to a predictable routine, died away and those of us who had no emergency rations did without until breakfast.

I had a few bandages and a humane killer, so they raked me in to deal with a few minor mishaps, but nobody was seriously hurt, nobody lost their tempers and nobody was disciplined. Perhaps Captain McNab wasn't such a bad Captain after all.

We had a rough couple of days in the Indian Ocean and one of the horses kicked the back out of its box but the ship's carpenter did a remarkable repair job between 2 and 4 a.m., leaving the box stronger than before, and the horse unharmed. I handed over the horses at the quayside in Singapore, had a few days touring the wonderful temples in Bangkok and flew home.

We caught one fly in the Red Sea. I sent it to the School of Tropical Medicine in Liverpool, but it wasn't the right kind to spread African Horse Sickness!

Bangkok Haircut

Eric and Maurice and I had three days to spare when we handed over our twenty horses in Singapore. The Ben Line's shipping agent, a charming Chinese Mrs Li, suggested that we should take the opportunity of visiting Bangkok and so, with amended tickets, we were collected by car and courier from the Ben Armin at 4 a.m. and were flying the Orchid air route an hour later.

The next two days were filled with river and waterway excursions to markets, temples, palaces and pagodas, a colourful fantasia in tropic heat made bearable by the water and the jungle shade: the whole visit pervaded by the charm and delicacy of the people, small, untiring and seeming perpetually young.

After weeks of peace aboard the ship, and the flesh pots (six regular meals a day, two Captain's conferences with liquid refreshment, and the engineers' galley to fend off any pangs of starvation on night tours of inspection) the Bangkok activity left me exhausted. At lunch time the two boys said they were going off with a couple of Americans. Our plane was to leave at 6 p.m. I took forty winks on my bed, packed my bag and paid the hotel bill. I thought I'd have my hair cut. The receptionist said the American (i.e. English speaking) barber was a taxi drive away but there was a good place round the corner.

The shop had only one chair in which a white coated young man was sprawled asleep. A girl was doing some book work behind the cash desk. She smiled as I came in and called to the barber who jumped up and swept me into the chair. The place smelled clean and hygienic and I thought I'd probably ask for a shave as well. The young man exchanged a few remarks with the girl and then there was silence. I realised that they were waiting for me. "Just a trim" I said. Silence. "Just a trim" I repeated and, glancing up in the mirror, saw their two faces and my own so solemnly poised on this ridiculous phrase that I laughed, said it again and made clipping gestures round the back of my neck. So,\ it was a joke! The barber and the girl laughed and chattered, explaining the joke to each other and to me and I tried to help with sympathetic smiles. Meanwhile they set about my haircut as a double act. I was settled back in the chair and was tucked in and raised and lowered and my hair was scissored and clipped and combed in a whirl of activity and chatter in which I was clearly included. The barber was swarthy and thick set. The girl was slim and pretty, probably half Chinese. They were taking a great interest in their work when another girl appeared. She was slimmer than the first and more delicately featured. While the barbering continued the phrase "just a trim" was explained to her with much laughter. She asked me "You like manicure?" My unenthusiastic "Well! I don't know" caused the girl such obvious disappointment that I smiled to reassure her. The effect was immediate. She laughed "You like! You like!" and started straight away on my hands.

The first girl produced a bottle for my inspection. I asked her for her name. From a long series of high pitched syllables, I selected Pimai for short. I had gathered that the young man was Rasa. The delicate beauty was Suree. The bottle Pimai was offering had VITAMIN LOTION AND TONIC printed on it and a picture of luxuriant hair. I nodded. This seemed to cause some concern so I nodded again and smiled. Happy laughter all round and lotion poured on my head. I was getting the hang of it. A solemn nod for "No", a happy nod "Yes". I tried an experimental smile on Suree. She laughed back and the others joined in. In case they might be jealous I was intending to repeat this with Rasa and Pimai but the opportunity had gone since Pimai was already piling hot towels on my face. Apparently, I was going to be shaved in any case. Rasa had tipped the chair back and was busy on the shampoo. Suree was making steady progress with my manicure. I decided I was in the hands of experts and settled down to enjoy myself.

The pitch of chatter fell and I relaxed while Rasa and Pimai, working neatly together, finished my shampoo, gave me the smoothest of shaves, trimmed my eyebrows and the hairs from my nostrils, and then did a very delicate spring cleaning job on my ears. Suree still had half one hand to do. Surely, they wouldn't leave her to work on alone. No! Rasa plugged in an electric vibrator and proceeded to massage my head, neck and shoulders. Then he put away the machine and worked thoroughly over the same area using his fingers and then the side of his hands in a noisy chopping action. The effect was a glow of positive well-being. Suree put the finishing touches to the last of my finger nails and then they were all responding to my smiling satisfaction with chatter and laughter. I said "Very good! That was very nice." And Suree asked "You like massage?" "Oh, yes" I said "I liked that very much!" Suree seemed pleased. She chirruped "You like! You like!" several times and disappeared through a side door. Rasa and Pimai stripped off my gown and stood me up to a similar chorus of "You like! You like!"

I reached for my wallet, but the idea was quite clearly conveyed to me that this was not the moment for settling up. I didn't want to offend them. Perhaps there was a tea ceremony or something. Then Suree's door opened to the sound of running water; steam was rising and I was being gently propelled in that direction. But I had had my massage! Then, with a sinking feeling I realised that massage might even include a bath. I really couldn't face any more. Any more what? So far, they had done nothing that was not thoroughly enjoyable and they were certainly efficient.

Suree had shed her overall and appeared from the steam in pale green shorts and a tight-fitting vest that showed her not quite as slim and delicate as I had thought. She looked so forlorn at the obvious reluctance of my approach that the least I could do was to smile at her. "You like, you like." Was her immediate response and, taking me by the hand, she drew me into her den. While Rasa and Pimai were helping me off with my clothes, Suree, with all the solemnity of a wine waiter, offered another bottle for my inspection. This too was labelled VITAMIN LOTION AND TONIC but the picture was not of luxuriant hair but of masses of bubbles. Relieved, I nodded solemnly but, quickly remembering my manners, added a beaming smile. The lotion was poured into the bath, there was some neat work with the towels and I was revelling in the hot water safely smothered in bubbles. Somebody was scrubbing me vigorously. I opened my eyes to look straight into Suree's dark brown ones and felt myself blushing in spite of the foam and her practical approach to the job in hand. "Sit down." She ordered. As I was lying on my back at the time, I was puzzled. "Sit down!" she said again and pulled me up into a sitting position. I corrected her with "Sit up!" and I lay down to show her what I meant. I decided to demonstrate the positions comprising the simple series, sit down, lie down, sit up and stand up; but realised that it would be futile to try and then, that it would be acutely embarrassing. I took time to lie back and enjoy the warmth and luxury of being bathed. Suddenly I remembered about catching the 'plane and, in a moment of panic, was going to ask for my watch but I was once again in demand. In such a surge of activity and laughter that I had no time to feel self-conscious, I was hauled out of the bath, well rubbed down and laid on a comfortable table for further processing. Suree set about me from the feet up. After nearly wrenching my toes out of their sockets she ran a finger across the sole of my foot. "Don't do that! I'm ticklish!" I yelled. Suree was delighted. She called Rasa and Pimai in. "He's tick-rish! He's Mr Tick-rish!" They had my name at last. This was very satisfactory and the new joke was added to their expanding vocabulary. Meanwhile Suree continued to subject each muscle, tendon and ligament to a sequence of rubbing, squeezing, pummelling and manipulation that I ceased to marvel at her strength and wondered ruefully about my own. She turned me onto my stomach and violently re-aligned my vertebrae, chop-chopped my shoulders and said "Sit down, Mr Tick-rish!" Dutifully, I sat up. Suree arranged me cross-legged on her table, flung open the door and presented her masterpiece, the refurbished Mr Tick-lish, to her admiring colleagues. The three chattered over their handiwork and the four of us were savouring the now classical jokes of "Just a trim, You-like, you-like and Mr Tick-rish, when Eric and Maurice peered in, backed out apologetically and then, realising who the central figure was in the tableau, blurted out, "Look here! We've got your bag in a taxi outside. Come on!" I would have been quite content to miss the 'plane but it turned out that there was no violent hurry. With as much dignity as I could muster, I hitched up my towel, climbed off the table, and introduced my friends. Pimai and Suree put their fingertips together to make little sloping roofs and bowed. Rasa helped me to dress while the girls produced cold drinks and made little welcoming speeches.

Once again, I produced my wallet but could get no clear indication from the resulting chatter of the amount of the bill. I chose a bottle of vitamin tonic and lotion, the bubbly one, as a souvenir, handed Rasa my last American Express order for ten dollars, bowed and finger-tipped ceremoniously along the line and was torn away by my oddly irritable companions. In the taxi, I discovered that it was not the time factor that was annoying them but the fact that they had spent a hot afternoon hunting for a massage parlour and had found that they didn't open until 6 o'clock!

We were joined on the aeroplane by one of the boys' American friends, Earl Ross. I was consciously content. I hadn't felt the comfort of bruised achievement since my rugger days and was aware of that flutter inside the ribs, the mutual greeting of a healthy body and an easy mind. Earl asked "What impressed you most, Sir, on your three days in Bangkok?" "Having my hair cut" I replied. Eric and Maurice, quite recovered from their pique, chuckled sympathetically. The American mulled it over for a few moments and then, with solemn politeness "Well", he said "I guess you English certainly have a sense of humour!"

Appendices

Curriculum Vitae

ALISTAIR C FRASER Major LVO, PhD, BVSc, MRCVS

Born 1903, Birkenhead

EDUCATIONAL BACKGROUND

1908-1913	Birkenhead Prep School
1911-1921	Birkenhead High School
1921-1927	Liverpool University
1927-1930	Cambridge University
	Ministry of Agriculture lab including 6 months at the Pasteur Institute in Paris (1930) and a trip to South Africa

PROFESSIONAL QUALIFICATIONS

Dec 1918	Junior Matric, Birkenhead School, age 15
July 1921	Liverpool University matriculation, age 18
Dec 1926	MRVCS, age 23
July 1927	BVSc, age 24
Nov 1930	PhD (Cantab), age 27

MILITARY CAREER

1914-1922	Birkenhead School Cadet Corps. Cheshire Regiment Rank: Lance Corporal
1922-1927	Liverpool University Territorials, Royal Lancashire Regiment Rank: Cadet
1927-1930	Cambridge University Royal Cambridge Regiment (Horses) Trooper
1940-1945	Royal Army Veterinary Corps, Lieut/Lieut.Colonel, Burma Star.

PUBLICATIONS

Fraser, Dr Alistair and Manolson, Dr Frank, Fraser's Horse Book, Pitman, 1979. This book was selected by jockey Bob Champion in 1988 as his favourite on Desert Island Discs.

Thear, Katie & Fraser, Dr. Alistair, The Complete Book of Raising Livestock and Poultry, Pan Macmillan, 1988.

Fraser, Alistair Cumming, A study of the blood of cattle and sheep in health and disease, University of Cambridge Thesis (PhD), 1930.

PROFESSIONAL APPOINTMENTS

1963   Honorary Veterinary Surgeon to HM the Queen

1966   Hon Member British Equine Veterinary Association (BEVA)

1973   Lieutenant of the Royal Victorian Order (LVO)

OCCUPATIONAL HISTORY

1910-1920   'seeing practice' as a young boy with uncles in practices in Wiltshire, Berkshire and South Wales aged 12-18 years.

1930-1933   Spilsby, Lincolnshire. Private Practice with Clifford Hall-Jones. Heavy horse. Practice on potato farms, declined due to arrival of mechanised transport.

1933-1938   Lambourn (Maddle Farm) and Aldbourne. Thoroughbred race horses, racing stables and stud farm partnership,

1940-1945   RAVC, Burma Star, Mule Training, Farriery Training. Retired as Major

1942   Mobile Veterinary Hospital, Burma.

1945-1956   Lambourn Veterinary Practice, Gill, Fraser & Bambridge

1956-1968   Wokingham Veterinary Practice, Fraser & Hopes

Retired to Aldbourne, Wiltshire.

Notes

[1] According to a cousin David Fraser's account, James Fraser took the ferry from Inverness to Banavie, then Fort William, then Glasgow. Thereafter, he took the boat from Glasgow to Liverpool, then train (his first experience of the railway) Liverpool to Wrexham. James' brother Alexander was already at Wrexham with Mr Cumming, the tea merchant and tailor, so probably Mary Cumming was his daughter. Details could be further explored via Denbighshire Archives who hold a large collection of family letters and papers lodged by another branch of the family as "Records of the Fraser Roberts family of Foxhall (1821-1979)".

[2] Duncan Cumming Fraser (1864-1952). Alistair's father attended Trinity Hall, Cambridge to read Mathematics, and became a prominent actuary who founded actuarial firm Duncan C. Fraser & Co., which continued until a merger with Mercer in 1986. Amongst other achievements, Duncan was actuary for the Titanic disaster relief fund and published on Newton's interpolation formulae.

[3] Sophie neé Storrar (1867-1941), she had attended Newnham College, Cambridge to read Natural Sciences. Sophie died in the blitz of 1941 on Birkenhead when their house was destroyed. Her husband Duncan survived the same bomb by sheltering under two upturned armchairs which he was ex-

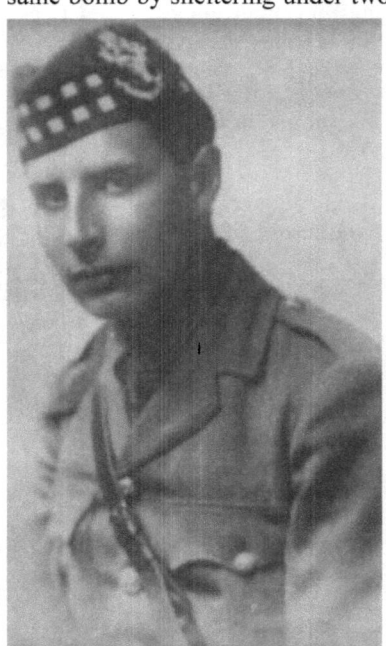

cavated from beneath in the cellar several hours later. All their papers, books and records were also destroyed.

[4] James Storrar (1832-1906), veterinary surgeon, m. Jean Morrison (1826-1917).

[5] James L. Fraser (1896-1919), known by his middle name Lesley, died from Tuberculosis while recovering from his war wounds. Birkenhead School's World War 1 memorial book gives the following account and image of Lesley:

James Lesley Fraser, eldest son of Duncan C Fraser, of Birkenhead was born June 1896 and died in Birkenhead on March 31st 1919. He entered the school in 1905, having previously been in the Preparatory and left in 1914, having been Head of the School in his last year and a member of the football XV. In the Corps he reached the position of sergeant. He left school to train for the army and after a few months with the Inns of Court O.T.C. obtained his commission. He first saw fighting in Mesopotamia, where he was wounded twice, in April 1916. He was invalided home for treatment for a wound in the knee which caused considerable trouble. While in hospital he unaccountably caught tuberculosis, from which he eventually died. His loss to the School is a very great one, for his loyalty as an Old Boy was above the ordinary. On one occasion when he was home on leave for three weeks he did not let a single day pass without putting in an appearance at the school. But it was for something more than his loyalty that he was beloved by all who knew him at the School. It was for his beautiful and strong character; for his transparent goodness, charm and kindliness. That the same opinion of him was formed where ever he went, is shown by all the letters received after his death. A brother officer wrote:- "He really was a fine chap. Absolutely one of the best fellows it has been my lot to meet, and I look back at my time spent with Lesley as amongst the happiest of days." His commanding officer wrote:- "He was a very good officer and I valued his services highly." A school-fellow wrote of him:- "Lesley was about the finest man I knew, fearless in upholding what he thought was right and he did good without making any fuss about it." While another said:- "I always used to think that Lesley must have had a good influence wherever he went, as he was so straightforward and strong willed and I know that in the army especially, it is the life a man leads and his actions that do more than any words and there is nothing more that men think more of than strong will for good things."

[6] Margaret (b. 1898) and Jean (b. 1909). Jean is not shown in the photos as they were taken around 1906 before she was born.

[7] David Storrar (1853-1938) and James Storrar (1858-1923)

[8] The friendship between Alistair and Clifford endured throughout their lives.

[9] Robert Barron m. Dora Lewis, in fact Alistair's first cousin once removed. Robert's father, Neil Barron (also a veterinary surgeon) had married Annie Storrar, Alistair's great aunt on his mother's side.

[10] Lieutenant-General Sir Michael Frederic Rimington, KCB, CVO, 1858-1928.

[11] The Army Remount Service was the body responsible for the purchase and training of horses and mules for the British Army between 1887 and 1942

[12] Charles Wentworth Elam MRCVS, DVH (1890-1966). Liverpool University Demonstrator in Veterinary Pathology and Parasitology 1916-1918, Part-

time Lecturer in Animal Management 1920-1955.

[13] This may be a mis-recollection of the identity of the staff member involved, or of the severity of the illness at that stage. According to the Liverpool University archives, Professor S.H. Gaiger was William Prescott Professor of the Care of Animals-Causation and Prevention of Disease at the Liverpool University Veterinary School from around this time in 1926-7 but did not die until 1934, years after Alistair had left. No similar name can be found during this time in the University staff records.

[14] Surra, a malarial-like infection in horses, caused by a trypanosome.

[15] Professor James Basil Buxton, M.A., D.V.M., F.R.C.V.S. (1888-1954), Professor of Animal Pathology, Principal and Dean of the Royal Veterinary College, Cambridge; President of the Royal College of Veterinary Surgeons, of the Central Veterinary Society, and of the National Veterinary Medical Association.

[16] Alistair rode his pony in the Cambridge Hunt races, without distinction we understand. We still have his racing silks.

[17] Professor Constantin Levaditi (1874-1954), born in Galati, dedicated to the therapy of syphilis, discovered and pioneered the use of the bismuth compounds as antisyphilitic drugs, and whose work led to the polio vaccine. He published more than 750 papers, won the "Paul Ehrlich" prize for chemotherapy (1931) and was elected Honorary Member of the Romanian Academy and Member of the French Medical Academy.

[18] It is suggested he may have had two beautiful daughters!

[19] At Alistair and Olive's Golden Wedding celebration in Aldbourne, Wiltshire, he re-affirmed his life's ambitions: to be a Veterinary Surgeon, to leave Merseyside and to marry a farmer's daughter. He had achieved them all by the age of thirty-five and declared himself to "have been coasting ever since"!

[20] Jullundur has changed name, and is now known as Jalandhar. The contemporary spelling has been preserved in the story.

[21] For his work 1940-1945 RAVC Mule training, Farriery training, and 1942 at the mobile Vet Hospital, Alistair was awarded the Burma Star. He retired as Major.

[22] Lieutenant-Colonel H.H. Shri Maharaja Sir Rajendra Prakash Bahadur, Maharaja of Sirmur, KCIE (1913-1964), last ruling Maharaja of Sirmur state.

[23] Lt Col. Sir John Miller (1919-2006). The Telegraph's obituary stated "A courtier through and through, Miller was effortlessly polite and wholly devoted to his Sovereign – though he was rather less genial to those whose social position was unclear to him."

Family Tree

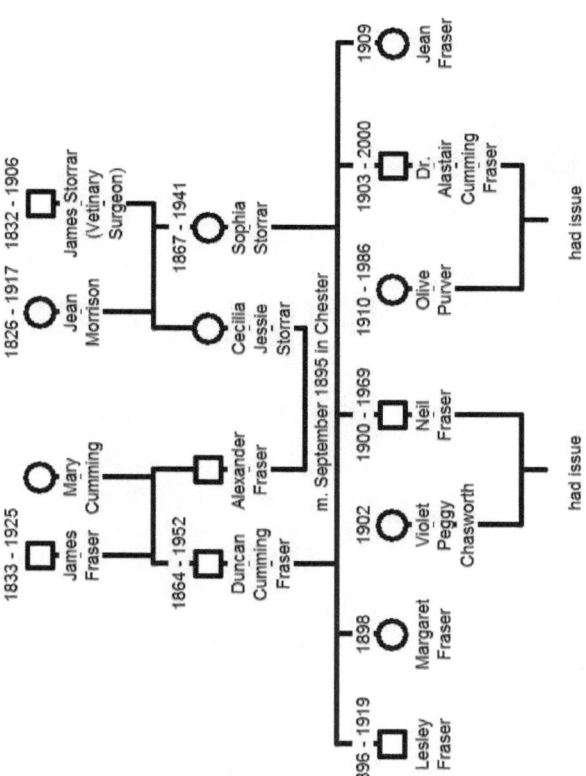

Alistair Fraser's grandparents, parents and their siblings

Index of Names and Places